Plant Based Meal Plan Cookbook

A Diet Plan with Tasty Vegan and Vegetarian Seasonal Recipes to Fix the Paradox of Healthy Eating and Have More Energy, a Better Nutrition, with a Weight Loss Solution

Steven MD Knives

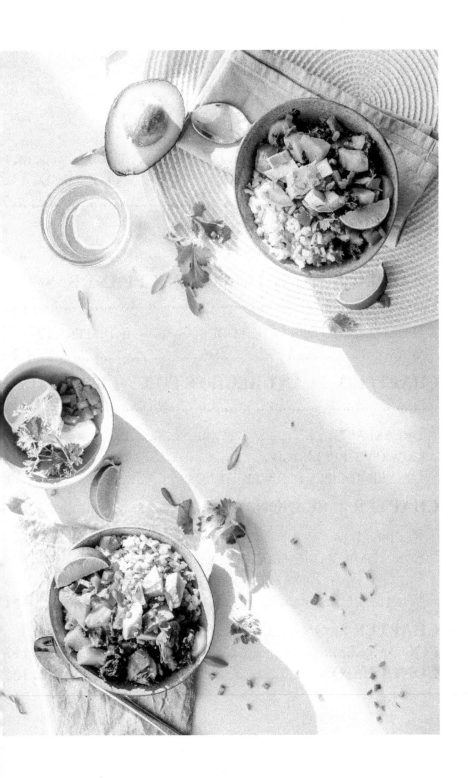

Table of contents

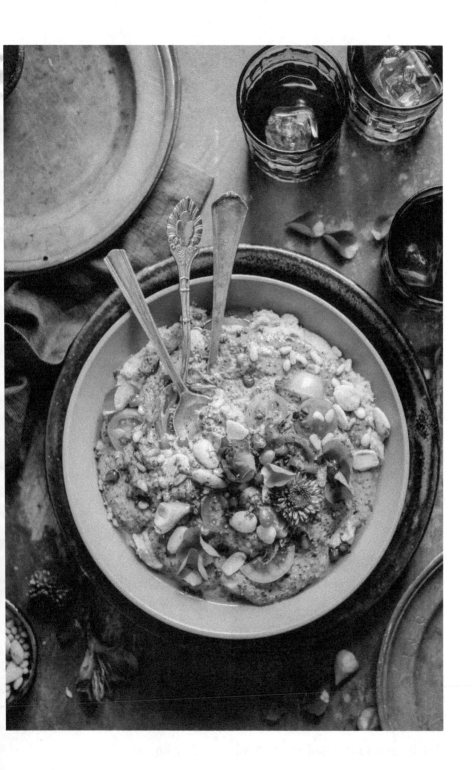

Introduction

Congratulations for choosing *Plant Based Meal Plan Cookbook; A Diet Plan with Tasty Vegan and Vegetarian Seasonal Recipes to Fix the Paradox of Healthy Eating and Have More Energy, a Better Nutrition, with a Weight Loss Solution* and thank you for doing so.

The following chapters give you an in-depth understanding of what entails a plant-based diet. You will find out the foods to eat and what to avoid while on this diet. The chapters also help you understand how plant foods can be useful for your weight challenges and even in preventing certain chronic illnesses associated with animal foods. Adapting to the plant-based diet is not easy for meat lovers. The chapters will help you in tailoring a smooth transition into the vegan way of life.

Through the chapters, you will find different plant-based recipes. There are outlined recipes for low calories that will help you keep your weight in check even without much trouble. The chapters have also provided for different seasonal recipes that are easy to make with the equipment you have at home. The book also includes guidelines on what items to purchase in the grocery store and the supermarket to help you develop and maintain a vegan lifestyle.

There are plenty of books on this subject on the market, thanks again for choosing this one! Every effort was made to ensure it is full of as much useful information as possible; please enjoy!

Chapter 1:

Understanding Plant Based Diet

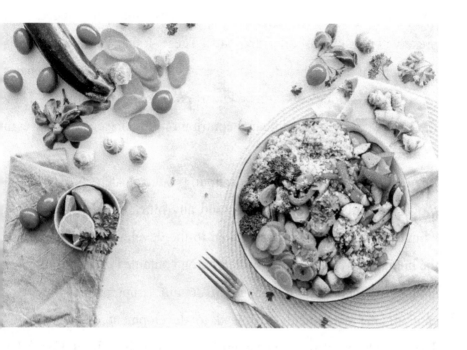

What entails a plant-based diet

The plant is a good source of closely all the nutrients required by the human body. Plant based diets include fruits, vegetables, nuts, whole grain, and legumes. These are basically plant based foods and whole foods. With the realization of the various health benefits attributed to plant proteins, people have shifted from consuming animal foods to plant-based foods. Plant based diet includes all unprocessed plant foods. It excludes the consumption of processed foods such as pasta and sugars. It excludes processed fruit juices, milk and milk products, all forms of meat (white and red), and eggs.

Foods to keep off when on a plant-based diet are as follows;

Avoid eating processed foods such as pasta and canned foods. Instead, go for fresh and whole foods. Processed foods are low in their fiber content; they also have other additives such as sugar, salt preservatives, excess oils, and fats. These foods are linked to the development of chronic illnesses such as cancer, diabetes, hypertension, kidney disease, and heart problems, among others. These foods are also a significant contributor to obesity and weight challenges.

Plant based diet excludes all animal products such as eggs, milk products, poultry, red meat, fish, and any other foods obtained from animals. Animal products are linked to the development of cancers in the human body, especially the heme iron contained in red meat. When animal products are cooked up to certain temperatures, they emit carcinogenic compounds that lead to development of cancer cells. These foods are also a major contributor to weight gain. Research has shown that it is rather a difficulty to watch weight while still on animal products. Animal related foods are also high in their fat contents and have zero fiber. Consumption of animal products leads to heart problems and hypertension as a result of clogged blood vessels. Their low fiber content makes it a cause of stomach problems such as indigestion and diarrhea.

Avoid the consumption of fast foods such as fries, burgers, cakes, ice cream, and pizza, among others. Fast foods have contents such as processed sugars and high sodium content, high fat content. These foods induce cravings in your body that lead to excessive eating and obesity. The foods are also very unhealthy as they contribute to increased risk of chronic illnesses such as cancer, hypertension, diabetes, heart problems, among others. Fast foods are also low in their nutrient content. Being addictive, when a person forms a habit of consuming fast foods, their bodies go low on some essential nutrients such as vitamins and minerals. They also contain additives that you do not want to put in your bodies due to their toxic nature.

Health benefits of plant diets

Plant foods offer a wide range of advantages over animal foods. They are scientifically recommended for healthy living as they promote a person's wellbeing. By eating plant-based foods, a person is able to reduce the risk of certain illnesses and avoid problems associated with overweight/obesity.

Plant foods are advantageous in their low fat and calorie load. They are also dense in their protein content. Proteins are excellent in helping a person watch weight as they prevent the gaining of body fat. By consuming plant proteins, a person produces more weight limiting hormones. Proteins also help in weight reduction by reducing the feelings of hunger while at the same time increasing the metabolic rate of the body.

By consuming plant products, a person reduces the risk of being overweight. Plants offer excellent sources of fiber, antioxidants, minerals, and vitamins. Plant foods are mainly high in fiber which is helpful in digestion as it limits the amount of sugars absorbed in the digestion process. The fiber in plant foods is also helpful in reducing cholesterol by preventing the absorption of fats in the foods we take. Fiber also helps in preventing constipation in enhancing the digestion of foods. It helps in the stimulation of the various digestive organs to produce important digestive juices. Enough intake of dietary fiber prolongs the amount of time food takes to move through the canal, increasing the absorption of minerals and vitamins in the food. It also prevents diarrhea and excessive hardening of stool.

Research has also confirmed that people who take foods high in fiber are at a lower risk of gaining weight. By consuming foods high in fiber, a person reduces the chances of developing type 2 diabetes. The reason behind the fiber preventing the occurrence of type 2 diabetes is the ability of the fiber to reduce the amounts of sugar the body absorbs maintaining a healthy blood sugar level.

It is also attributed to lowered cholesterol and reduced risk of developing heart disease. The fiber in the digestive system also clumps fats reducing the rate at which they are digested and absorbed in the body. Healthy bacteria in the gut thrive on soluble fiber. The bacteria microbiome feeds on the remains of fermented fiber in the digestive system. These bacteria help in the production of short-chain fatty-acids that help in reducing cholesterol in the body. The short chain fatty-acids also promote good health by reducing inflammation in the body. Inflammation is a risky condition linked to the development of serious illnesses such as cancer among others.

Plant foods reduce the risk of cancers, such as colorectal cancer. While animal foods are found to increase the risk of cancer, plants contain phytochemicals and antioxidants that reduce the risk of developing cancer while at the same time fighting the progress of cancer cells. The fiber found in plant foods is also helpful in detoxification of the body. The detoxification process is aided by both soluble and insoluble fiber. The soluble fiber absorbs the excess hormones and toxins within the body, preventing them from being taken up by the cells. Insoluble fiber works by preventing the absorptions of toxins fond in the foods we consume from the digestive track. It also increases the time which food takes to go through the digestive track. The process is said to reduce the body's demands for more food. The soluble fiber also stimulates the production of certain components that reduce the feelings of hunger which include peptide YY, peptide-1, and cholecystokinin.

When a person is on a plant-based diet, they cut on their consumption of processed foods and refined sugars that are harmful to the body. These sugars promote weight gain by increased food cravings and the production of certain hormones that induce the body to crave for food. These sugars and other additives found in processed food also increase the risk of cancer and among other illnesses.

Plant foods are also rich in certain components that are found to possess anti-oxidation properties while also working in reducing cholesterol levels in the body. These components are polyphenols, such as flavonoids, stilbenoids, and lignans. For instance, green tea, which is most commonly used for its anti-oxidation properties is rich in (epigallocatechin gallate) a flavonoid responsible for the production of the fat burning hormone.

11

Another beauty of eating plant foods is that you worry less about overeating. The plant foods contain limited calories and negligible levels of harmful fats. According to research, persons who eat plant foods live longer as compared to those that feed on animal foods. Plants foods not only improve the quality of life by protecting a person from illnesses but also lower the risk of early deaths resulting from these illnesses and health conditions.

Plant based foods are also friendly to the environment. Eating plant foods encourages the planting of more plants to give more foods that protect the ozone layer by absorbing excess harmful carbon dioxide from the atmosphere. Plants based diet discourages the industrial practices associated with processing foods. These practices promote the release of harmful gases into the atmosphere, and the packaging of the foods makes use of materials that are not environmentally friendly.

Chapter 2:

What to Eat on a Plant Based Diet

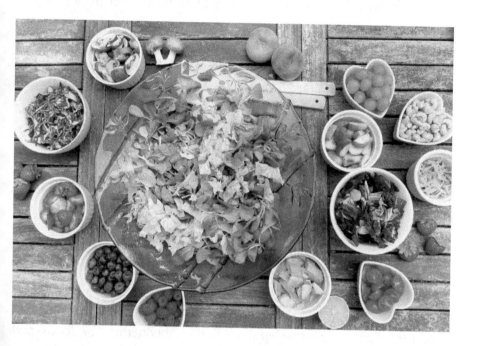

Plant based foods include but not limited to the following;

- Fruits (limiting processed fruit juices and squeezed out juices)
- Fresh vegetables
- Nuts
- Whole grains like barley, quinoa, oats and brown rice among others
- Legumes; such as beans, peanuts, lentils, chickpeas, and peas.
- Seeds
- Unsweetened beverages
- Spices and herbs

- Plant based oils
- Plant proteins such as tempeh and tofu

Shifting from a less focused diet to a plant-based diet in not easy at first, but it is manageable. Here are several tips helpful in achieving a full transformation to a plant-based diet:

Start slow and avoid pressuring yourself too much about the diet. Start slowly by taking unsweetened tea. Limit your intake of animal proteins, cut down on processed foods, and avoid eating junk foods. Find substitutes for animal products such as milk and meat.

Maximize on vegetable soups and plant-based salads. Make it a habit of eating a plateful of salad and bowl full of thick plant soup before meals. It will reduce your appetite for food and also boost your plant foods intake.

Stock your kitchen with plant-based foods. Avoid shopping for animal products. Apply the same strategies when budgeting for foods and planning meals for guests and other people living in your house. Having certain animal products in your home will tempt you to eat them. Avoid stocking junk and processed foods in your home as it will also increase your cravings and lure you to eating them.

Aim at starting your day with a breakfast based on plant foods. Make this your habit and make your breakfast fun by including foods you enjoy most. Resist the temptation to include certain foods deemed ideal for breakfast such as bacon, sausages, chicken wings, eggs, among others.

Throughout the day, keep plant-based snacks at hand. You can take out your own home prepared seeds, nuts, and salads to work. It will limit the temptation to eat any foods that come your way when the body sugar levels go down.

Make vegetable part of your main meal. Eat vegetables as much as you can. When cooking, make a point of using health friendly oils of plant origin such as peanut, sesame, canola and olive oil.

It is essential to be aware and conscious of the foods you are, including in our diet. Take note of your previous habits and check out foods that are not plant based; those that are plant based but processed and canned foods and make a conscious decision to avoid them. Be strict in avoiding these foods as they are the most likely cause of stagnating in your adaptation of the plant-based diet.

When deciding on what to cook, make your meals fun and enjoyable. Try out different exotic plant-based recipes. Avoid cooking foods that you do not enjoy eating as a desperate move to assume a plant-based diet. Make the transition experience as exciting as possible by planning meals around ingredients and components that are affordable and readily available.

When stating up on this new diet, avoid being too hard on yourself whenever you go against it. Set achievable timelines and plan on the way to go about it by laying out procedural steps. At the same time, avoid giving it too much time as the transformation stage might turn into a lifestyle. Be strict on what you plan out to do and be cautious of pitfalls.

In making the diet easier to adapt, try to educate your family and close friends on what it entails and its significance to a person's health. Having the people, you live with, and friends you closely interact with aboard will help you stay focused. It will also prevent the frequent temptation to go back to the harmful foods you are trying to avoid.

Ingredients for plant foods as per the different seasons

Summer foods

Zucchini, water melon, tomatoes, tomatillos, summer squash, strawberries, raspberries, plums, peaches, okra, mangoes, limes, lima beans, lemons, honeydew melons, green beans, garlic, eggplant, cucumbers, corn, cherries, celery, carrots, cantaloupe, blueberries, blackberries, bell peppers, beets, bananas, avocados, apricots, and apples.

Winter foods

Winter squash, turnips, Swiss chard, yams, sweet potatoes, pineapples, pears, parsnips, oranges, onions, limes, lemons, leeks, kiwi fruit, kale, grapefruit, collard greens, celery, carrots, cabbage, Brussels sprouts, beets, bananas, avocados, and apples.

Spring foods

Turnips, Swiss chard, strawberries, spinach, rhubarb, radishes, pineapples, peas, onions, mushrooms, limes, lettuce, lemons, kiwi fruit, kale, garlic, collard greens, celery, carrots, cabbage, broccoli, bananas, avocados, asparagus, apricots, and apples.

Fall foods

Winter squash, turnips, Swiss chard, yams, sweet potatoes, spinach, rutabagas, raspberries, radishes, pumpkins, potatoes, pineapples, peas, pears, parsnips, onions, mushrooms, mangoes, limes, lettuce, lemons, kiwi fruit, kale, green beans, grapes, ginger, garlic, cranberries, collard greens, celery, cauliflower, carrots, cabbage, Brussels sprouts, broccoli, bell peppers, beets, bananas and apples.

Chapter 3:

Plant Recipes for Weight Loss

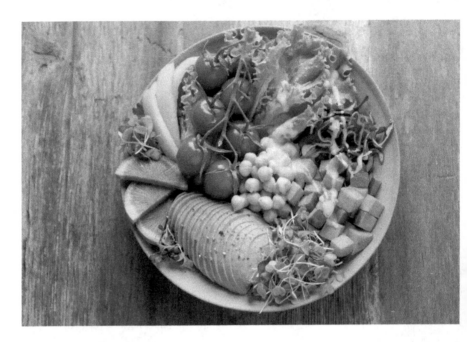

We will be looking at recipes for persons interested in reducing their weight and those watching their weight. We are going to look at light foods that are low in fat content and whole foods. To achieve a lower calorie and low-fat diet, go easy on nuts and seeds, increase your intake of fruits, vegetables, grains, legumes, and beans.

Breakfast

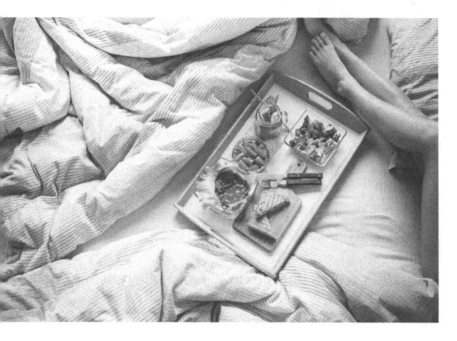

Here are some options you could be looking at for breakfast;

Ayurvedic oatmeal

Ingredients

- Half teaspoon of turmeric powder or alternatively pealed and rasped curcuma/turmeric 20mm
- A pinch of ground cloves and a quarter teaspoon of cardamom
- Two sticks of cinnamon
- 10 ounces of soy milk
- 80 grams of Oatmeal flakes
- 1.5 table spoon of raisins
- 1.5 table spoon of pumpkin seeds

- Sliced fresh pumpkin 0.2kgs
- 7 ounces of tap water

Method

Boil the shredded pumpkin in water in low heat till soft and well done.

Put in the soy milk then bring the mixture to boil once again.

Include the turmeric, cardamom powder, cinnamon sticks, and the oatmeal in the mixture.

Let the food cook for 10minutes.

Include the pumpkin seeds by sprinkling them in the dish.

It is now ready to serve.

Cantaloupe with dates oatmeal and mint-melon relish

Ingredients

- A pinch of salt
- A quarter cup of quick cook steel-cut oats
- A quarter cup of coconut milk
- A quarter tsp of coconut oil
- Two pitted and chopped dates
- A cupful of cantaloupe cut in cubes and a separate half cup of the same.
- One tsp of mince mint leaves
- Two blackberries, preferably fresh

Method

Puree the coconut oil, dates and cantaloupe in a food processor.

Pour the puree in a pan and add the coconut milk and simmer the mixture.

Include salt and oats and simmer.

As the moisture simmers, start on the mint-melon relish.

Slice the blackberries and cantaloupe into a quarter inch sized pieces.

With fresh mint, toss the blackberries and cantaloupe mixture.

Put the cooked oatmeal in a bowl once it is cooked to your satisfaction.

Add the mint-melon relish on top of the oatmeal and splash some coconut milk over the dish.

Granola bars

Ingredients

- Melted dark chocolate
- A teaspoonful of almond extract
- One third glassful of organic coconut oil
- Half glass of pure maple syrup
- Half glass of pure natural almond butter
- Three quarters of teaspoon sea salt
- A teaspoonful of Ceylon cinnamon
- Two table spoonsful of chia seeds
- Two table spoonful of shelled hemp seeds
- A quarter cupful of natural desiccated coconut
- A half cupful of raw pumpkin seeds
- Half cupful of raw sunflower seeds
- Half cup of roughly chopped natural raw walnuts

- A cupful of dried cherries that have been presoaked and drained
- A cupful of roughly chopped raw almonds
- Two and a half cups of rolled old fashioned gluten free oats

Method

Line your oven with a standard parchment cookie sheet and preheat to 325F.

Mix the salt, cinnamon, chia seeds, hemp seeds, coconut, pumpkin seeds, sunflower seeds, walnuts, the presoaked cherries, almonds, and oats, in a bowl and put aside.

In low heat and in a small pot, put the coconut oil, almond butter, and the maple syrup. Keep stirring as it melts. Remove from the heat and mix in the almond extract.

To the dry ingredients, you had set aside, add the wet mixture, and keep mixing until satisfied with the outcome.

Firmly on the baking sheet, press the granola in a layer and make it spread evenly.

In the preheated oven, let it cook for a maximum of 30 minutes then remove it and let it cool down.

Once cold, cut into pieces of your liking.

Drizzle the pieces with the melted chocolate.

Oatmeal with apricot

Ingredients

- Six tablespoonfuls of either maple syrup or agave nectar

- Two cupful of any non-dairy milk of choice
- A half teaspoonful of salt
- One teaspoon of ginger (ground)
- One and a half teaspoon of baking powder
- Four tablespoons of ground flaxseeds
- Three cupful of rolled oats
- A cupful of water
- One and a half cups of chopped dried apricots.

Method

Prepare an 8-inch baking pan and pre heat your oven to 375F.

Cover the chopped apricots in hot water and let them soak for 10 minutes and let them retain the water.

Mix salt, ginger, baking powder, flaxseeds, and the rolled oats, and put them aside.

Mix the soaked apricots with the agave nectar and the milk. Put this mixture in to the oatmeal and stir till it becomes even.

In a baking pan, spoon the mixture and bake for 35 minutes.

Let it cool for 15minutes and serve.

Alternatively, you can split it into pieces of your preferred size when cooled and keep refrigerated.

Banana dates flux sugar free muffins

Ingredients

- A half cupful of chocolate chips, the semi-sweet vegan type.
- A cupful of chopped pecans

- A half cupful of unsweetened coco nut flakes
- Half teaspoon of stevia in powder form
- Half teaspoon of baking soda
- Half teaspoon of baking powder
- A quarter teaspoon of allspice
- A quarter teaspoon of cardamom
- A teaspoonful of cinnamon
- Half teaspoon of salt
- A quarter cupful of brown rice flour
- A quarter cupful of barley four
- A quarter cupful of flaxseed meal
- A cupful of whole wheat pastry flour
- Two teaspoons of vanilla extract
- A quarter of non dairy milk of choice
- A quarter cup of tahini
- A quarter cup of date paste
- Two ripe bananas

Method

Oil ten muffin tins and preheat the oven to a temperature of 350F

Mash the ripe bananas in a bowl and mix in the vanilla extract, milk, tahini, and the date paste.

In a separate larger bowl, whisk the stevia, baking soda, baking powder, allspice, cardamom, cinnamon, salt, brown rice flour, barley flour, flaxseed meal, and the whole wheat pastry flour.

Stir in together the dry and wet ingredients until they are evenly mixed. Then mix in the chocolate chips, pecans, and the coconut and stir the mixture.

In the baking tins, scrape in the mixture and bake for half an hour.

Let the cooked muffins slightly cool then remove them from the tins and place them on a rack to cool completely.

Oil and sugar free mango lime pancakes with coconut and ginger

Ingredients

- Two divided mangoes
- One tablespoon of chopped crystallized ginger
- One tablespoonful of grated fresh ginger
- A quarter teaspoon of natural lime extract
- Zest from one lime
- Juice extract from one lime
- One tablespoonful of apple cedar vinegar in nut milk or two cups of butter milk
- A quarter teaspoon of cinnamon
- Two teaspoons of baking soda
- One teaspoon of baking powder
- To tablespoons of wheat germ
- A quarter cup of unsweetened coconut flakes
- A quarter cup of coconut flour
- A quarter cup of macadamia nuts

- One and a half cups of whole wheat pastry flour

Method

Heat a skillet or a griddle. Crank your oven to 200F with the breakfast plates inside.

Mash or process the macadamia nuts into little pieces and place them aside.

Peel one half of the mangoes and cut into small pieces.

Peel the other mangoes, mix with lime juice and blend them to a smooth consistency.

On a separate clean bowl, mix the spices, baking soda, baking powder, wheat germ, coconut flakes, and coconut flour. When done mix in the macadamia pieces.

In another bowl, whisk the lime extract, lime zest, and buttermilk. Include the lime and mango mixture and stir. With a whisker, mix this mixture with the dry ingredients. Include the mango pieces and mix. Add both the crystalized and fresh ginger and let the mixture sit for 20minutes.

Spoon the mixture on to the hot skillet and sprinkle oil on its surface (optional).

When the pancakes bubble on the surface and seize to shine, flip them and let them cook for a few minutes.

Put them in the preheated oven to prevent them from going cold.

You can serve them with the syrup of your choice

Pomegranate quinoa porridge

Ingredients

- Coconut flakes for garnishing
- Stewed apples
- A quarter cup of desiccated coconut
- One pomegranate pulp
- Ten pitted organic prunes and cut into quarters
- One teaspoonful of vanilla extract
- Two and a half teaspoons of cinnamon
- Three capfuls of almond milk
- One and a half cups of quinoa flakes

Method

Stewed apples

Cut the peeled apples in to pieces

In a sauce pan with water, cook the apples in low heat till they soften.

Then remove them from the water and mash them

The porridge

In a sauce pan, place the almond milk and quinoa and cook under low heat for 8 min. keep stirring till the mixture attains even consistence.

Include the vanilla extract, the desiccated coconut and cinnamon in the mixture and taste as you add to achieve your desired taste.

Pit prunes and divide into thirds and add into the mixture and stir.

Serve the porridge in separate bowls and add the stewed apples

Mexican frittata (oil-free)

Ingredients

- A quarter cup of chopped cilantro
- One and a half cups of black beans
- One teaspoon of old bay seasoning
- Six thinly sliced small potatoes
- One seeded and cut redbell pepper
- One tablespoon of Dijon mustard
- One teaspoon of sea salt
- One and a half teaspoon of granulated garlic
- Three tablespoonfuls of nutritional yeast
- A quarter cup of arrow root or corn starch
- Two boxes of mori nu tofu

Method

Preheat your oven to 375F

Grease an eight-inch pan

Blend together the mustard, onion powder, garlic powder, salt, corn starch, nutritional yeast and tofu in a blender until it is smoothly done. Put the mixture in a mixing bowl and keep adding the old bay seasoning till the combination takes your desired speckled appearance.

Include the half of the cilantro, put the black beans and bell peppers and mix.

In a pre-set baking dish, let it bake until it takes a gold-brown color (roughly should take 45mins)

When ready, serve with the sauce of your choice.

Mexican chocolate waffles

Ingredients

- One teaspoon of vanilla extract
- Three table spoons of water and one able spoon of flaxseed meal thoroughly mixed and let for some minutes
- Four ounces of natural apple sauce
- Hundred and twelve ounces of Mexican lager
- One teaspoon of stevia in powder
- A quarter teaspoon of salt
- A quarter teaspoon of chipotle chili powder
- A teaspoon of cinnamon
- A half teaspoon of baking soda
- One and a half teaspoon of baking powder
- Half cup of unsweetened cocoa powder
- A cup and three quarters of whole wheat pastry flour

Method

Let an open bottle of beer sit in the fridge while open over night

At 2ooF put the diner plates in the oven.

Sprinkle some oil on to the waffle iron and heat it.

Mix the stevia, salt, chili powder, cinnamon, baking soda, baking powder and cocoa powder in a larger bowl.

With the flat beer, mix the flaxseed meal, vanilla extract, and the applesauce. Add this mixture into the dry one and combine till evenly done.

In the hot waffle iron, pour in the batter to a closely filled up level.

Cook till crispy and see to it that it disengages from the iron with ease.

Repeat the procedure for the remaining waffles.

Banana bread muffins

Ingredients

- Two tsp of pure maple syrup
- Half tsp of vanilla extract
- Half cup of mashed ripe banana
- Two tsp of vegan chocolate chips
- A quarter tsp of cinnamon
- Half tsp of baking powder
- A half cupful of whole oats and an extra two tbsp.
- A half cup of oats flour

Method

Prepare 4 muffin tins by spraying with non-sticky spray.

Preheat oven to 360F.

Process half cupful of oats till it forms even flour.

Mix the dry ingredients in a bowl setting aside the chocolate chips.

In a bowl, add and mix the mashed banana, together with the dry and wet ingredients.

Include the chocolate chips in the mixture and stir.

Scoop the mixture into the muffin tins and cook in the preheated oven for 13minutes.

When done, cool it for a few minutes.

You can keep it in a tightly closed container for up to 2 days.

Stracciatella muffins (for serving 12 people)

Ingredients

- Five ounces of finely grated chocolate or vegan chocolate chips
- Two tbsp. of oil
- Half tbsp. of salt
- One pack of baking soda
- Two packages of vanilla sugar
- Three quarters ounces of brown sugar
- Eight and a half ounces of flour
- One tbsp. of vinegar
- A cupful of soy milk

Method

Preheat the oven to 355F

Add the vinegar to the soymilk and mix

In a larger bowl, include the salt, baking powder, vanilla sugar, and flour and mix till well done.

Add the soy milk and oil into the mixture and mix using a spoon.

Fold in the chocolate chips.

Bake the dough in the tins till it no longer sticks to a toothpick when pulled out (that is for approximately twenty minutes)

Chocolate chip banana bread

Ingredients

- Dairy free chocolate chips
- Half tsp of nutmeg
- Half tsp of ground cinnamon
- Three cups of self-rising flour
- Three fifths cups of dairy free milk
- A cup of golden castor sugar
- Three cups of ripe bananas

Method

Line your baking tin with grease roof paper.

Preheat oven to 360F.

Mash the ripe peeled bananas in a bowl to paste.

Put in ground nutmeg, ground cinnamon, milk, and the sugar and mix well.

In three stages, fold in the flour till well done.

Include the chocolate chips by folding them in too.

Put the paste into the lined tins.

Include extra chocolate chips on the surface.

Bake it for seventy minutes.

Zucchini bread with pistachios and fennel

Ingredients

- A quarter cup of raw chopped pistachios
- Three tbsps. of coconut oil
- One tbsp. of apple cedar vinegar
- A quarter cup of plan dairy free yoghurt
- Two tsps. of fennel seeds
- Half tsp of salt
- One tsp of baking soda
- One tsp of baking powder
- A quarter cup of tapioca starch
- A half cup of almond flour
- Three quarter cups of brown rice flour
- A cup of quinoa flour
- A cupful of sugar
- Six tsps. of hot water
- Two tsp of ground flax seeds
- A pond of yellow summer squash and zucchinis

Method

Line the bottom of a four and a half inch by eight-and-a-half-inch loaf pan with flour

Pre-heat oven to 350F

Using the larger holes of the grater, shred the yellow squash and zucchini and let the mixture drain in a strainer for half an hour.

While the mixture drains, combine the hot water with the falx seeds and set it aside to slur.

Dry the zucchinis mixture in paper towels by squeezing it. In a bowl, mix it with apple cedar vinegar, and the plain yoghurt

Whisk the coconut oil together with the sugar in a mixing bowl. Include the flux slurry and combine it.

Combine half of the zucchini with half of the flour mixture keep adding both as you mix until you finish both mixtures.

Into the baking pan include the batter and top it with the remainder of the pistachios and let it bake for one hour. Cool it for a quarter of an hour before moving it into a cooling rack.

You can have it warm or let it cool completely, alternatively let it sit in the fridge overnight to flavor and eat it in a maximum of two days.

Zucchini quinoa peas pancakes

Ingredients (for ten pancakes)

- A quarter tsp of salt
- A tbsp. of salt
- Half cup of quinoa flour
- A tsp of olive oil
- A tbsp. of vanilla extract
- Two ripe bananas
- A whole zucchini
- A cupful of green peas

Method

Process the olive oil, vanilla extract, bananas, zucchini and the green peas in a food processor.

Thoroughly mix the salt, baking powder and quinoa flour in a bowl.

Combine the zucchini mixture with the flour mixture

Heat and grease a non-sticky pan

Cook by spooning one and a half teaspoons of the mixture in to the pan into a circular shape.

When well done on one side, flip and cook the other. Repeating this process for the whole batter.

Banana chocolate chip muffins

Ingredients

- 2.47 oz of chocolate chips
- Two tbsp. of caramel extract
- 1.4oz sunflower oil
- 5. oz of ripe bananas
- 6.35 oz of the nondairy milk of choice
- Half tsp of baking powder
- 3.5 oz of sugar
- 9.17 oz of self-rising flour

Method

Combine the flour and baking powder in a bowl

Preheat oven to 356F

Combine the oil and milk in a bowl and whip it thoroughly. Include the sugar in the oil/milk mixture and combine well.

Combine the mixture well.

Mash the bananas and include them in the wet mixture.

Combine with the flour by including it in portions as you mix till all the flour is gone.

Include the chocolate chips in the mixture.

For 60minutes bake the mixture in muffin tins until golden.

To see if they are ready, test them using a toothpick. It the dough doesn't cramp on the toothpick stick; they are ready to serve.

Cardamom persimmon scones with maple persimmon cream

Maple cream

- A quarter tsp of salt
- A quarter tsp of cinnamon
- A tbsp. of maple syrup
- Three quarter cup of non dairy milk
- Two tbsps. of shredded coconut
- Half cup of persimmons chopped

Scones

The wet ingredients

- A cupful of chopped Fuyu persimmons.
- A tsp of vanilla extract

- A teaspoon of apple cedar vinegar
- Half cup of almond milk
- A cupful of plain vegan yoghurt

The dry ingredients

- Three table spoons of soft coconut oil
- Half tbsp. of salt
- Half tbsp. of cinnamon
- A tsp of cardamom
- Two tsps. of baking powder
- A tbsp. of coconut sugar
- Two cups of all-purpose flour

Method for preparing the cream

Blend all the cream ingredients in a blender

Good with the scones when warm.

You can have it in the fridge for up to 2 days

Method for the scones

Line a baking sheet on the oven with parchment. Preheat oven to 400F. Put together the salt, spices, baking soda, sugar, and flour in a mixing bowl. Mix the components evenly. Add coconut oil into the mixture. Whisk the vanilla, apple cedar vinegar, almond milk, and yoghurt in a bowl. Carefully mix in the dry and wet ingredients till well combined without overdoing it.

Using a wooden spoon, fold in the chopping's of persimmons.

O a flat firm surface, sprinkle some flour and bring the dough into a round shape of not more than an inch thickness.

Divide it into eight wedges separate wedges and transfer them into the preset baking sheet.

Let them cook for a maximum of 20 minutes and let it cool down.

It is now ready to serve along with the cream.

Quinoa crepes

Ingredients

- Vegan butter oil or if you prefer, Coconut oil spray
- Two tsps. Of vanilla extract
- Three tbsps. of maple syrup
- One and a half tbsp. of ground flax seeds
- Four and a half cups of almond milk
- Three cups of quinoa flour

Method

If your flax seeds are not ground, grind them in a blender (highspeed)

Whisk the ingredients together in a bowl till they smoothen.

On medium heat in a crepe pan, heat some coconut oil.

Let your pan heat up first.

Apply a thin layer of the batter on your pan in a round shape.

Cook until a brown color appears on the edges.

When its easily coming off the pan, flip on the other side and let it cook as well.

Do the same for the remaining batter.

You can serve with the topping of your choice. Try out vegan Nutella and fresh berries if you like.

Coconut brown rice dressed in avocado cream

Ingredients

- Coconut oil to roast
- One tbsp of roasted pine nuts
- One celery stalk
- Half cup of black beans (rinsed and drained)
- An orange sweet potato
- One and a half cup of coconut crème
- One and a half cups of water
- Two cups of brown rice

Avocado cream ingredients

- Paprika
- Pepper and Salt to taste
- Dash of quality olive oil
- Grated ginger of 20mm
- Two tbsp. of coconut cream
- Half lemon juice
- An avocado

Method for preparing the Avocado cream

Blend together the coconut cream, ginger, lemon juice and avocado in a blender till the cream smoothens. As you blend, add olive oil sparingly.

Keep scraping off the blender sides till you arrive at the desired consistency.

Add the seasoning of pepper and salt.

Best served chilled.

Method for preparing brown rice

Roast the cube-shaped sweet potatoes in coconut oil until they soften.

In a pot, put in the presoaked brown rice and include the coconut cream and water. Bring the content to boil.

When it boils, reduce the heat. Let it cook in a low heat or simmer. Keep watch to keep it from burning. Let the rice take in all the water and don't rinse off.

If you prefer, make use of a rice cooker.

Slightly roast the pine nuts and chop the deveined celery.

When cooked, mix in the rice with the celery and beans in a bowl, and add salt for seasoning.

Include the avocado crème, roasted potatoes topping with the pine nuts.

Buckwheat and coconut porridge with Blueberry sauce

Ingredients for the porridge

- Half tsp of vanilla essence
- Half tsp of cinnamon

- Two tbsps. of coconut oil
- Two dates or alternatively two tbsp. of rice malt syrup
- Half cup of coconut milk
- One and a half cups of buckwheat (soaked and rinsed)

Ingredients for the blueberry sauce

- Four tbsp. of coconut water or natural water
- One tbsp. of rice malt syrup
- One cupful of blueberries (unfrozen)

Ingredients for topping

- One banana
- Roasted coconut flakes

Method

Put together all the ingredients for making the porridge and blend. When it smoothens, transfer into a bowl.

In a clean blender, blend together the ingredients for the blueberry sauce. Make it easier to blend by adding on some water but don't put too much water.

With a spoon swirl the blueberry sauce on to the porridge.

Include your toppings.

Buckwheat and hempseed pancakes

Ingredients

- For the ginger-lemon syrup

- One tbsp. of lemon zest
- One-inch ginger
- One cupful of maple syrup

Ingredients for making the pancake

- Coconut oil for cooking
- One and a half tsps. of vanilla extract
- A pinch tsp of salt
- A quarter tsp of baking soda
- One and a half tsps. of baking powder
- Two tbsps. of ground flax seeds
- Three tbsps. of hemp seeds
- Four medjool dates
- A cupful of non-dairy milk of choice
- A cupful of raw buckwheat groats

Method for pancakes

Soak the buckwheat groats in water and make sure the water covers them entirely and rises above them by a few millimeters. Squeeze in lemon juice and let them sit overnight.

Strain off the water and rinse off the groats. Let the water drain off completely.

If you are using dry dates, let them soften in hot water for some time and drain the water off.

Over medium heat, preheat a nonstick skillet. In a high-speed blender process together with all the ingredients till they smoothen.

On the sauce pan, put a half teaspoon of the coconut oil. Pour on the mixture right from the blender. Use two tablespoons for each.

When the edges start detaching and the top bubbles, flip our pancake to cook the on the other side. Repeat the same procedure for all the pancakes. The pancakes will have a dark appearance.

As you cook put the pancakes on a diner plate in a warm oven of 200F.

Method for preparing the lemon ginger syrup

In a pot, including the lemon zest, slices of ginger and the maple syrup.

Let them cook over low heat for five minutes.

Turn down the heat and leave it for ten minutes.

Strain the syrup.

Protein pancakes

Ingredients

- Cooking coconut oil
- A pinch of sea salt
- One tsp of melted coconut oil
- Half cup of almond milk
- One tsp of baking powder
- One mashed banana
- a scoop of vegan protein powder

Method

In a bowl put together the milk, melted coconut oil and mashed banana and mix.

Include the salt and baking powder in the mixture.

Mix in the protein powder as you keep stirring until you arrive at a desirable consistency.

Melt the coconut oil in a non-sticky pan over low heat.

When well heated, spread a thin layer of the mixture on the surface and cook till it bubbles on the surface. Flip over when cooked and cook the other side until it is well done.

Do so for the remaining mixture.

You can include your favorite toppings as you serve.

Quinoa and oats focaccia bread

Ingredients

- A quarter cup of olive oil
- Half cup of quinoa flakes
- Half cup of oat flour
- Two cups of gluten free wheat flour
- One tbsp. of psyllium husk
- One tsp of sea salt
- One tbsp. of maple syrup
- Five tsps. of active dry yeast
- Two cups of lukewarm water

Method

In the warm water, let the yeast dissolve.

In the dissolved yeast, include the psyllium, maple syrup, and salt and combine.

Mix in the quinoa flakes and the flours and stir well.

Add the oil into e mixture and combine once again.

Leave the mixture covered in a dump cloth through the night.

The following morning put the dough into a baking tray and brush on some oil.

Preheat your oven to 350F.

Oil and flour your hands and do the flour in to the desired focaccia shape, making it thin.

Leave the bread to rise and make some holes in it. Put some generous amounts of oil into the holes.

Include rosemary, and cherry tomatoes on top and let it bake for twenty minutes till it turns golden brown on the surface.

Sweet molasses bread

Ingredients

- Old fashioned rolled oats
- Three half tsp of instant yeast
- One and a quarter tsp of salt
- Half tsp of ground nutmeg
- Two tbsp of brown sugar
- Three tbsp of unsweetened cocoa powder
- Two and two-thirds of white whole wheat flour

- Three cups of all-purpose wheat flour
- Four tbsp of coconut oil or non-dairy butter
- Half cup of molasses
- Three half cups of warm non dairy milk or almond milk

Method of preparation

Put together all the dry ingredients plus the yeast and combine them.

Using a wooden spoon, mix in the butter, molasses, and milk. When mixed in, use your hand side to knee the mixture to a smoother texture. Covered in a kitchen clothe, let the dough rise in a warm place for about 60 minutes.

Dust a flat surface and places the dough on it. Split it into three equal portions and give them the shape of bread.

Place the dough pieces in greased baking tins, or greased baking sheets. Alternatively, use a parchment lined baking sheet.

Sprinkle on oats and leave it to rise while covered for another 60 minutes.

As it rises, preheat your oven to 350F.

Cook for 30 minutes and test if it is well done using a toothpick or a tester. The color should deepen when cooled.

Remove the pieces of cooked bread and place them on a rack to let them cool.

You can have them cooled or while still warm.

Low calorie lunch

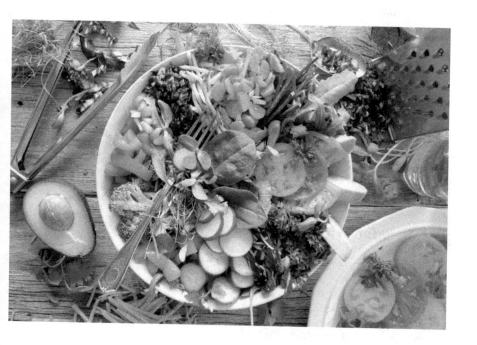

Kales salad with oranges and fresh figs

Dressing ingredients

- Stevia and agave
- One teaspoon of cinnamon
- Half teaspoon of Himalayan salt
- One juiced organic orange
- One Avocado

Salad ingredients

- Two peeled and deseeded organic oranges split into chunks

- Nine dried and Soaked or fresh organic figs divided into quarters free of the stem
- A bunch of organic kales. Chopped free of stalks
- Chopped organic parsley (handful)

Method

Mash all the dressing ingredients in a bowl as you mix. Include parsley and kales to the dressing and used your hands to breaks them down and combine. Top with figs and oranges.

Potato salad with chickpeas spinach

Salad ingredients

- Olive oil cooking spray
- A handful of fresh spinach
- Two Chopped cremini mushrooms
- One tbsp of chopped red onions
- A quarter cup of chopped bell pepper
- A quaternary cup of cooked chickpeas
- Medium sized potato unpeeled and cubed into half inched pieces

Ingredients for the spices

- Pepper and salt to taste
- A pinch of cayenne
- A quarter tsp of paprika
- A quarter tsp of ground cumin

- A table spoon of chopped fresh basil leaves
- Half tsp of chopped fresh rosemary leaves

Method

Spray a heavy cooking pan with oil. Heat the pan over medium heat.

Place the potatoes on the pan and spray over them. Make sure they are evenly distributed and cover the pan.

Cook the potatoes for 10 minutes or till they form a crust on their surface.

Chop the mushrooms, bell pepper and onions.

When cooked, put in the chickpeas and replace the lid for another two minutes.

Add salt, mushrooms, bell peppers and onions, putting aside the basil leaves. Cook for another two minutes as you stir.

Include the spinach leaves and stir till they wilt and remove the pan from the heat. Sprinkle on the chopped basil leaves and serve immediately.

Lentil barley soup with potatoes

Spice ingredients

- Pepper and salt
- Half tbsp of turmeric
- Half tbsp of fenugreek
- Half tbsp of paprika
- A tbsp of Cummins

Soup ingredients

- Seven cups of water or low sodium vegetable broth
- A can of diced tomatoes
- Two cups of cubed potatoes half inch size
- One third cup brown rice or alternatively dry barley
- Half cup of diced lentils
- Three minced garlic cloves
- One chopped celery rib
- One peeled and chopped carrot
- One chopped medium sized onion

Method

Include a heavy bottomed soup pot, pour in two tbsp of vegetable broth or water. When it begins bubbling, include the garlic, carrots, celery, and onions. Cook the vegetables under medium heat till they soften. This should take approximately five minutes. Stir as you cook and add more water or broth if necessary.

Let the water or broth boil in a separate pot.

Include the spices and remaining ingredients to the vegetables, leaving aside the pepper and salt. Stir in the food and pour in the boiling water or broth. Once it boils, reduce the heat and place a lid cover the soup. Leave it for half an hour to endure the barley, lentils, and potatoes are well cooked.

Put in the pepper and salt, and taste. When satisfied with the seasoning, let the soup stand for a few minutes to cook then garnish it with your favorite greens.

Lentil soup with mushrooms

Ingredients

- Two tbsp off nutritional yeast
- four cups of vegetable broth
- A package of sliced cremini mushrooms
- Three chopped carrots
- A quarter cup of small red lentils
- A cup of green lentils
- Two Bay leaves
- Two grinds of pink salt
- Black pepper (generous grinds)
- Half tsp of cumin
- Two minced garlic cloves
- One diced small onion
- A tsp of olive oil

Method

Place a pot on medium heat. Fry the onions in the pink salt and olive oil for 60 seconds. Include salt, pepper, Cummins, and garlic and let it cook for another 60 seconds. Add the vegetable broth, bay leaves, and the green lentils. Let the mixture boil while covered. Cook until the lentils are well cooked and soft for about twenty minutes and bring down the heat. Cook it under low heat for five minutes.

Include the mushrooms, carrots, and red lentils. Cook under simmered mode till they are all cooked.

Remove for the heat and include the nutritional yeast and stir. Let the soup sit for ten minutes or more or less for the flavors to meddle. Alternatively, you can serve it right away.

Sprouted mung salad

Ingredients

- Salt
- A quarter cup of finely chopped coriander leaves
- A tsp of sugar
- Juice of half a lemon
- Two teaspoons of garam masala
- A quarter teaspoon of turmeric powder
- Two teaspoons of coriander powder
- Two minced garlic cloves
- Two slits green chilies
- One finely diced tomato
- A thinly sliced medium onion
- A teaspoon of vegetable oil
- A cup of dry mung beans

Method

Heat the oil in a large saucepan

Sauté in the onions with salt until they assume a brownish color

Put in the red chilies and garlic and cook for a moment

Add the cumin powder, turmeric coriander, and tomatoes and stir. Cook till the tomatoes partly soft.

Mix in the sprouted mung beans. Let them cook under low heat for a quarter hour while covered. Let the beans assume your desired cooked texture. You can add water and stir them as they cook.

When cooked, add the lemon juice, sugar, and salt. Finally, include the coriander and serve.

Root vegetable soup

Ingredients

- Freshly ground pepper
- A can of cannellini beans (rinsed and drained)
- Two spoonsful of Italian seasoning
- Two tsp of organic tamari
- Two minced garlic cloves
- A sliced onion
- A sliced celery bunches
- A cup of sliced green beans
- Eight Oz of sliced cremini mushrooms
- Three sweet potatoes peeled and sliced into cubes
- Five peeled and sliced carrots
- Five (peeled and cut into cubes) russet potatoes
- Two cups of water
- 65oz of vegetable broth

Method

With enough water covering the vegetables put all the vegetables in a pot and bring to boil. Reduce the heat but keep the vegetables boiling. Simmer the pot and cook for one hour.

Remove the pot from the heat and let it sit for 10 minutes. Serve while still warm. It goes well with crusty whole bread.

Turmeric chickpea soup

Ingredients

- Soy yoghurt
- Pepper and salt
- Half vegetable stock cube
- Water
- Two cups of rinsed and drained chickpeas
- A quarter teaspoon of ground cumin
- Half teaspoon of garam masala
- Half teaspoon of paprika
- A teaspoon of ground turmeric
- A thumb size minced fresh ginger
- Two minced garlic cloves
- One diced onion
- A tablespoon of olive oil

Method

Fry the onions in olive oil in a pot for a few seconds. Include ginger and garlic and cook till they release a fragrance. Put in the spices. Include the peas and stir to cover them in the mixture.

Pour in some water till the food is fully covered the cover the pot and let it boil.

Include the stock cube in the soup while still boiling then mix and simmer.

Let is cook under low heat for half an hour.

Add pepper and salt and taste.

Put the cooked soup in a blender and blend it till it goes smoothly.

Transfer the soup to a bowl and sprinkle some soy yoghurt.

It is now ready.

Vegetable croquettes and couscous

Sauce Ingredients

- Pistachios
- Water
- Extra Virginia oil
- Sweet paprika
- Basil
- Rocket

Croquettes ingredients

- Durum wheat (re-milled)
- Untreated whole sea salt

- Pepper
- Extra-virgin oil
- One tsp of lemon juice
- One tbsp of pitted black olives
- Three tbsp of cornmeal flour
- Two tbsp of rice starch
- Two sage leaves
- Six basil leaves
- Six mint leaves
- Two-inch leek
- A white cauliflower
- Two carrots
- 3.5oz of whole couscous

Method for preparing sauce

Put a tablespoonful of iced water, paprika, basil, and Rocket into an immersed mixer and blend together.

Include the oil and Pistachios and continue to blend to achieve complete smoothness in the sauce.

Sprinkle the sauce on the croquettes while they are still warm

Method for preparing croquettes

Follow the manufacturer's instructions in preparing the couscous

Blend together the olives, sage, mint, basil, peeled carrots, leek and cauliflower. Into the mixture, put virgin olive oil, pepper, and salt. Blend till it goes smooth.

Pour the mixture into a bowl. Include the cornmeal flour, starch, and couscous. To thicken the mixture, put in a tbsp of durum wheat semolina.

Use a pastry cutter to make croquettes of 1.5-inch diameter on a baking sheet lined with parchment paper. Make croquettes of the whole mixture.

Cook under 400F in a ventilated oven till they achieve a brownish color.

Greens and seeds kaniwa salad

Ingredients for dressing

- Salt
- Three lemons juice
- Two mashed garlic cloves
- Two tbsp of olive oil

Ingredients for the salad

- A quarter cup of chopped chives
- A quarter cup of chopped dill
- Tsp of poppy seeds
- Three tbsp of pumpkin seeds roasted and salted
- Three tbsp of sunflower seeds roasted and salted
- Two tbsp of Chia seeds
- Two tbsp of sesame seeds roasted
- A quarter cup of kaniwa

- Two handfuls of arugulas
- An avocado
- A cup of diced raw zucchini
- Half a cup of fresh peas
- A cup of blanched and sliced asparagus

Method

Boil kaniwa in a pot with a half cup of water. Add a quarter tsp of salt. When boiled, simmer down the heat and cook till the water is soaked up.

Dissolve some salt in water and bring it to boil. While boiling, put in the peas and asparagus. Let it boil for three minutes and remove them from the water and slice them.

Put together the poppy seeds, sesame seeds, Chia seeds, pumpkin seeds, sunflower seeds, peas, asparagus, zucchini, and kaniwa seeds, and mix in a bowl.

Cut the chives and dill into pieces and include them in the bowl.

Mix the minced garlic, lemon juice and olive oil, and pour over the mixture. Add some salt to taste.

Mix the salad evenly and garnish with the avocado slices.

Serve over any greens of your choice.

Detox salad

Dressing ingredients

- Salt
- A quarter cup of unfiltered apple cedar vinegar
- Half cup of olive oil
- Three garlic cloves

Salad ingredients

- Two third cups of chopped walnuts
- Half cup of fresh drill
- One avocado
- One red beet
- Six carrots
- A small-sized green or red cabbage

Method

Process beets, carrots, and shredded cabbage in a food processor and transfer the mixture into a bowl

Roughly process the walnuts separately.

Mix up the pressed garlic cloves, vinegar and oil to make the dressing for the salad.

Not the vegetables, add some salt, walnuts and the fresh drill. Include the dressing on the vegetables and combine the mixture. Taste and add more salt and vinegar if need be and let the Salas sit for fifteen minutes.

Add the chopped avocado on top and sprinkle some of the walnuts. Ready to serve.

Potato pierogis, sauerkraut and wild garlic with sour creme

Ingredients for the stuffing

- A pinch of white pepper
- Half tbsp of nutmeg
- Half tbsp of apple cedar vinegar
- A quarter tsp of sea salt
- A tbsp of nutritional yeast
- Half cup of sauerkraut
- Three boiled medium sized potatoes
- Three tbsp of vegan sour cream

Ingredients for toppings

- Four tbsp of vegan sour cream
- Two red onions

Ingredients for the dough

- A quarter tsp of sea salt
- Three tbsp of wild garlic Pesaro
- A cupful of water
- Three cups full service of all-purpose wheat flour

Method for preparing the stuffing

Boil the potatoes in water till they soften. Put them in a bowl and add the sour cream.

In the bowl, include white pepper, nutritional yeast, apple cedar vinegar, nutmeg, and salt. Combine the mixture as you mash in the potatoes. Include the sauerkraut and keep mixing.

Bring the dough out of the refrigerator and use your hands to massage it. Sprinkle some flour on it and roll it thin. Use a glass to do round shapes off the dough. Further, make each circle into an oval shape by pulling with both hands.

Put a teaspoon of the mixture in the middle. Bring the opposite edges together and press on them to close. Do the same till you are through.

Caramelize onion rings in a pan

On the side, heat salted water in a pot and include the pierogis. Once every they come to the surface, put them in a pan over medium heat. Cook them until they turn golden on the edges.

Serve with sour crème and the onions on top.

Method for preparing the dough

Using a wooden spoon, roughly stir together water, wild garlic Pesto, salting, and the flour. Use your hands to press on the mixture until it is well combined. When done, let it sit in the fridge in an oiled bowl for a while.

Quinoa onigirazu sushi sandwich

Ingredients for the miso ginger sauce

- A cup of water
- A tbsp of apple cedar vinegar
- Two tbsp of maple syrup or coconut nectar
- A tbsp of coconut amino
- One lime juiced
- Two pieces of peeled ginger root
- Three tbsp of miso
- Two tbsp of tahini

Ingredients for the filling

- A handful of fresh cilantros
- A leaf of Swiss chard
- Half cup of pickled, roasted or cooked beet
- Half Avocado
- A shredded carrot
- A quarter sliced English cucumber

Ingredients for turmeric quinoa

- A quarter tsp of salt
- A quarter tsp of black pepper
- Half tsp of tsp of turmeric powder
- A cup of water
- Half cup of quinoa

Ingredients for the onigirazu (two organic nori sheets)

Method for the turmeric quinoa

Under running, tap rinse the quinoa on a sieve and let the water completely drain off

In a saucepan, mix in salt, pepper, turmeric, water, and the quinoa. Let the mixture boil under medium to low then simmer to allow the quinoa to take in all the water.

Take it from the heat and let it sit for five minutes then fluff with a fork.

Method for the miso ginger sauce

Include some water and blend together all the sauce ingredients as listed. Use a high-speed blender and blend till the contents are smooth.

Bring the two together:

On a clean kitchen counter, lay out the nori sheets with the shinning side under. You can have it on a clingy sheet.

Place a quarter portion of the quinoa in the middle off the sheet and make it flat.

Include the vegetables on top. That is the cilantro, cucumber, beet, carrot, avocado, and chard. Let the vegetables spill over and cover with another quarter piece of quinoa.

Wrap the quinoa using the nori sheets as a package. You can make the edges meet in the middle.

Use the clingy wrap to seal by covering over tightly. Turn the upper side down and leave it for five minutes. Apply the same procedure for the rest. Use the miso sauce as an accompaniment. You can split the sandwich in to two using a wetted sharp knife.

Don't let it go over 24 hours.

Quinoa lentil salad with roasted egg plant

Dressing ingredients

- Three tbsp of lemon juice
- Pepper and salt
- Three tbsp of pine nuts
- Two mandatory half oz of finely chopped onions
- Two garlic cloves
- Six tbsp of olive oil
- Three tbsp of nutritional yeast
- Eighty-eight Oz of basil

Ingredients for the salad

- Garlic powder
- Salt and pepper
- Two tbsp of olive oil
- Two and a half Oz of chopped sun-dried tomatoes
- Eighteen Oz of eggplant cubes
- Five Oz of quinoa
- Five Oz of beluga lentils

Method

Separately boil the quinoa and lentils.

Let the eggplant chops sit in salty water for thirty minutes. Drain off the water and wash them then put them in a bowl. Add garlic powder, pepper, salt and two tbsp of oil.

Preheat oven to 350F and bake the mixture in a baking pan. Make sure it is evenly spread.

Once it begins to brown, take them out and allow them to cool.

Separately blend the pepper, salt, nutritional yeast, oil, pine nuts, garlic, and basil.

Mix the eggplants, onions, sun-dried tomatoes and lentils in a bowl. Include the quinoa and mix well. Add the pesto and keep mixing. If need be, adjust the seasoning by adding more salt or pepper or both. Sprinkle the mixture with the extra nutritional yeast.

You can have it warm or cold, depending on your preferences.

Whole wheat pizza crust

Ingredients

- A cup of all purpose
- Half cup of whole wheat flour
- Half cup of semolina wheat flour
- A tbsp of sea salt
- 2 tbsp of olive oils
- A cupful of water
- A cupful of active starter

Method

Mix in the same salt, olive oil, the cup of water, and active starter together. Include the flour in bits till you achieve a soft dough. Make use of all the flour. Cover the mixture in a clean wet cloth and let it sit in a warm place for 24 hours.

Uncover the dough and use your hands to press on it and fold it. Leave it has the refrigerator for at least ten hours, but the longer you leave it, the better it gets.

To start on the cooking process, preheat your oven on the highest temperatures. On a floured board, divide the dough into halves and put the vegetables of your choice on top. Let the food cook in the oven for at least twelve minutes.

You can have your pizza warm or cold.

Kales salad with peanut sauce

Ingredients

- Three tbsp of chopped oil free peanuts
- A tsp of hot sauce
- A tsp of ginger powder
- Two tsp of minced garlic/ two garlic cloves
- A tbsp of freshly squeezed lime juice
- One and a half tsp of soy sauce or tamari
- Half cup of water
- Half cup of natural peanut butter with no deities
- A peeled red onion split into half
- Four chopped medium carrots
- Four cups of chopped kales or any other leafy green you prefer

Method

Lightly blend the onions and carrot chunks. In a bowl combine the mixture with the kales.

In a food processor, pour in the hot-sauce, ginger, garlic, lime juice, tamari, water, and peanut butter. Blend the mixture to a smoother paste. In the bowl, toss the paste along with the vegetables. Sprinkle on a tsp of chopped peanut.

Fennel brown rice salad

Ingredients

- A tbsp of tahini
- Brown rice
- Hummus
- A handful of baby tomatoes
- Two cups of baby spinach
- A red bell pepper
- A tbsp of apple cedar vinegar
- One lime
- One fennel bulb

Method

Chop off the two ends of the fennel bulb

Divide vertically into halves and wash them in a bowl or water and vinegar. Alternatively, if you are using organic fennel bulb, rinse thoroughly under running water.

Slice the building into thin pieces. In a bowl combine the slices with the lime juice, apple cedar vinegar, and the baby spinach. Once well mixed allow the flavors to sink in for half an hour.

Chop the baby tomatoes and the bell pepper and include them in the marinated salad. Add Hummus as you serve and have it with brown rice. You can increase the calcium content in the rice by drizzling on some tahini.

If need be, add more seasoning; that is pepper and salt.

Dinner recipes for weight loss

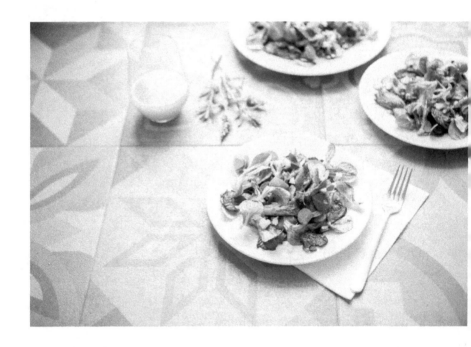

Kale soup, white bean and winter potatoes

Ingredients

- Freshly cracked pepper
- Sea salt
- Three handfuls of chopped kales

- Two tsp of thyme
- Two tbsp of nutritional yeast
- Four cups of vegetable broth
- A handful of chopped sun-dried tomatoes
- A can of cannellini beans (rinsed and drained)
- Two minced garlic cloves
- A diced onion
- A tbsp of olive oil or sesame oil
- Diced blue/purple potatoes
- A diced sweet potato

Method

Heat the oil in a pot and put the potatoes. Let them cook for a few minutes over low heat then add the garlic and onions. Cook as you stir till, they assume a brownish color.

In the pot, include the sun-dried tomatoes, beans, nutritional yeast, and the broth. While covered, let the pot boil over medium heat then reduce the heat to a simmer. Cook till the potatoes are well done them turn off the heat and add the kales. Stir them while the content is still hot.

Ready to serve. Top the dish with almond parmesan and cracked pepper. It goes well with crusty bread.

Dill soup, spring kales with rice

Ingredients

- Lemon wedges
- Half cup of fresh chopped drill
- Freshly ground black pepper and salt
- A can of small butter beans
- Four Oz of baby kales detached from the stems
- Six cups of vegetable broth
- Four minced garlic cloves
- Five thinly sliced carrots
- Half cup of arborio rice
- A quarter tsp of chili flakes
- One minced red onion or three minced spring onions
- A tbsp of neutral oil

Method

Heat oil in a pot and fry in the chili and onions till they soften. In the pot, include the garlic, carrots and the rice.

Add the pepper and salt to the food for seasoning and let them cook for a minute.

Include kales, beans, and the broth and bring to boil. Once boiled, reduce the heat and simmer to allow it to cook. For brown rice, you will need to give it more time to cook.

Finally, add the drill and stir. If need be, add more chili and seasoning. Serve with the lemon wedges.

Lentil soup and lemon

Ingredients

- Freshly squeezed lemon juice
- Freshly chopped cilantro
- Freshly ground black pepper
- A tsp of paprika
- A tsp of ground coriander
- One and a half cups of rinsed and drained red lentils
- Two cups of chopped carrots
- Three minced garlic cloves
- Two cups of freshly chopped onions
- Six cups of low sodium vegetable broth

Method

Pour in the vegetable broth into a saucepan.

Add the freshly ground pepper, paprika, coriander, minced garlic, and the sliced onions. Let the food boil while open for a few minutes as you stir occasionally.

Include the red lentils and cook for a further fifteen minutes. Put in the carrot chopping and cook while covered till the lentils are well prepared. Stir the food and lower the heat if need be to prevent it from burning.

Garnish with fresh cilantro and half freshly cut lemon.

Black bean chili and Chipotle sweet potatoes

Ingredients

- Water
- A quarter tsp of smoked paprika
- Two tsp of ground cumin
- Two tbsp of ground chili
- One and a half cups of rinsed and drained black beans
- 13oz of undrained diced tomatoes
- One and a half pounds of peeled and half an inch diced sweet potatoes
- Two minced garlic cloves
- A cup of diced green pepper
- A cupful of diced yellow onions
- Two dried chipotle chilies

Method

Add the Chipotle chilies in hot water and let them soak for sixty minutes to soften. Cut them into pieces.

In a cooking pot cook the pepper and onions in a few teaspoons of water till they start to brown. Include the chopped chipotle and the minced garlic and let them cook for a minute.

Include sweet potatoes, cumin, and chili powder and cook as you stir. Make sure the potatoes are well covered in the spices. Let them cook for five minutes them pour in the tomatoes.

Use the Chipotle along with the water and include them in the mixture. Allow the food to boil covered. Once boiled, reduce the heat to a simmer making sure the food is still raging. Cook till the sweet potatoes soften. It should take about half an hour.

When cooked, include the beans and add more seasoning if needed. Include the paprika and let the food cook for another ten minutes.

It goes well with sprouted bread, but you can have it with the grains of your choice.

Date, tempeh and olive Marbella

Ingredients

- Enough brown rice for four
- 10 Oz of fresh greens
- A half cup of dry white wine
- Half cup of freshly squeezed orange juice
- Half cup craters with juice
- A quarter cup of chopped kalamata olives
- A quarter cup of chopped green olives
- A half cup of chopped pitted dates
- A tbsp of water
- A tbsp of tamari
- Half cup of vegetable broth
- A quarter cup of red wine vinegar
- 2 tbsp of dried oregano
- Eleven minced garlic cloves

- Eight Oz pack of tempeh split in half

Method

Bring the two halves of tempeh to boil in water in a medium sized pan. When boiled reduce the heat to a simmer and give it ten minutes. When softened drain of the water and let it cool down.

In a baking pan, include the black pepper, capers, olive, dates, water, tamari, vegetables broth, red wine vinegar, oregano and minced garlic. Mix in the ingredients and add sliced pieces of the tempeh. Stir the food and make sure it is evenly combined.

Refrigerate the food while covered overnight. When set to start cooking, preheat the oven to 350F. Pour in the white and the orange juice with the food.

Let it bake it in the oven for 60 to 90 minutes. Stir up the food severally as you bake.

If need be added more broth to the baking food, steam the vegetables on the side. Prepare your rice to go along. Serve the tempeh with the cooked vegetables and rice.

Garnish the food with orange and parsley.

Raw pizza

Crust Ingredients

- A quarter cup of walnuts
- Two bell peppers
- Two dates
- One garlic clove

- Half onion
- Freshly squeezed juice of half a lemon
- Two tomatoes
- Three zucchinis

Sauce Ingredients

- A garlic clove
- A date
- A handful of fresh basil leaves
- Freshly squeezed juice of half a lemon
- Half cup of chopped zucchini
- Half cup of sun-dried tomatoes

Topping ingredients

- A tsp of apple cedar vinegar
- A bell pepper
- Two cups of mushrooms
- Two tomatoes

Method

Using a spiral slicer, to slice the zucchini into noodles. Blend the rest of the crust ingredients without adding the zucchini noodles. Pour the smoothly blended mixture in with the zucchini noodles in a bowl. Spread a thick layer of the zucchini mixture on a dehydrator or tray. State your oven at 115F. It should cook for six hours. Keep checking and flip on to cook the other side once one side is done. It should come off pliable.

For the sauce, blend together all the sauce ingredients until they turn smooth and pour evenly on the cooked crust.

Slice the vegetables thinly, spray on the apple cedar vinegar and let them dehydrate in the oven to soften for forty minutes. Place the toppings on top of the pizza and slice it into pieces.

Black bean buggers (until-free)

Ingredients

- Whole wheat buns
- Instant oats
- Pepper, salt and cayenne
- Half tsp of dried oregano
- A tbsp of ground cumin
- A quarter minced fresh cilantro
- 15 Oz of rinsed and drained black beans

Method

Preheat your oven to 350F.

Blend the black beans in a processor until well mashed.

In a bowl, mix the mashed beans with the spices and the cilantro. Include a quarter cup of oats and mix well to reduce the stickiness. Place the mixture in the fridge for ten minutes. Divide the dough into three pieces and model them into patties. Place them on a greased cookie-sheet lined with parchment paper and bake for seven minutes in the preheated oven. Flip it and spray the other side and let it cook for another seven minutes.

Best served warm.

Vegan Lobster rolls

Ingredients

- Lemon wedges
- Vegan butter
- Hoagie rolls 26 inch
- A quarter cup of vegan mayonnaise
- A quarter tsp of lemon juice
- Two tsp of old bay seasoning
- A tsp of minced garlic
- Half cup of chopped onions
- A quarter cup of red bell pepper dices
- A quarter cup of chopped celery
- A can of hearts of palm
- Two and half tbsp of grape seed oil

Method

In a skillet, heat two tbsp of oil and cook in the hearts of palm for ten minutes. Stir as you cook to prevent them from sticking to the pan. Remove from heat when they brown on both sides and let them cool down.

Add pepper and celery and combine them. Sauté onions in a half tsp of oil on a skillet over medium heat. Add garlic once every they translucent and cook for a minute. Turn off the heat and combine the sautéed onions with the hearts of palm. Mix and include mayo, lemon juice and old bay seasoning to the mixture.

Toast the hoagie rolls and apply butter on the inner sides. Serve the hearts of palm on the rolls and garnish with lemon wedges.

Kales edamame Hummus (oil free)

Ingredients

- Salt
- A quarter tsp of smoked paprika
- A tsp of black pepper
- A tsp of garlic powder
- A tsp of green chili sauce
- A tbsp of liquid amino
- Six tbsp of water
- One and half lemons' juice
- A quarter cup of tahini
- Three minced garlic cloves
- A cupful of chopped kales
- A cup of frozen edamame (thaw and drained off)
- A can of rinsed and drained garbanzo beans

Method

Put together all the ingredients and process to smoothen in a food processor. Include some more water if need be.

Stuffed squash lentil curry

Ingredients

- A handful of chopped fresh coriander
- A tbsp of balsamic vinegar
- A quarter tsp of sugar
- Two tbsp of olive oil
- Pepper and salt
- A quarter tsp of ground ginger
- A quarter tsp of cinnamon
- A Half tsp of garam masala
- A tsp of curry powder
- A handful of dry chopped apricots
- A handful of chopped walnuts
- Five chestnut mushrooms
- Two minced garlic cloves
- Half finely diced onion
- A packet of black lentils
- Half butternut squash

Ingredients for tahini drizzle

- Two tbsp of water
- A tbsp of tahini

Method

Cut the butternut squash into two equal parts from head to tail and remove the seeds.

Preheat your oven to 350F

Sprinkle on some olive oil and let it cook on a baking sheet in the oven for fifty minutes till it softens. Scoop the squash and leave thirty millimeters flesh in it. Put the scooped squash aside.

On a frying pan add a tbsp of olive oil and cook in the garlic till it assumes a brownish color then put in the onions and let them cook to translucent.

Include sugar, spices, all the herbs, nuts, lentils, mushrooms and put a few tips of water. Add the chopped apricots when the mushrooms are well done. Include the scooped squash in the mixture and mix.

Pour in the mixture into the squash and sprinkle with balsamic vinegar. Grill the stuffed squash for five minutes.

Method for preparing the tahini

Put a cup of water in a bowl and stir in the tahini. Sprinkle of the mixture on the stuffed squash and the chopped coriander on top.

Now ready to serve.

Jackfruit sandwiches

Ingredients for the sandwich

- Two tbsp of vegan butter
- Dill pickle slices
- Eight slices of vegan ham
- Eight slices of vegan cheese

- Yellow mustard
- Four Cuban rolls

Ingredients for the jackfruit

- Two cans of rinsed and drained jackfruit
- Ground black pepper
- A tsp of salt
- A tsp of ground cumin
- Two tsp of onion powder
- A tbsp of chopped cilantro
- Three minced garlic cloves
- Two tbsp of tamari
- Three tbsp of maple syrup
- A quarter cup of vegan mayonnaise
- A quarter cup of lime juice
- A quarter cup of orange juice

Method for preparing jackfruit

Line your oven with a baking sheet with parchment and preheat to 375F.

In a bowl includes pepper, salt, cumin, onion powder, cilantro, garlic, tamari, mayonnaise syrup, lime juice, and orange juice, and whisk them together.

Chopped the jackfruit in a food processor. Include a bowl, mix it with the marinade. Bake it in the preset oven for half an hour.

Method of preparing the sandwich

Half the bread and apply mustard on both sides. Place cheese on the bottom and top of the bread. Line it with jackfruit, pickles, and ham.

In a heavy pan cook the sandwiches in medium heat in preheated oil. Cover the pan with another heavy pan and press on the sandwiches as they cook. You could put something relatively heavy on top of the covering pan.

Cook the sandwiches while pressed for five minutes. Ensure the cheese is melted, the bread toasted, and sandwich flattened. An electric panini grill would serve you well. If you have one, you can make use of it.

Divide the sandwiches into halves and enjoy while still warm.

Jackfruit wraps

Ingredients

- Olive oil
- Pepper and salt
- Six roti
- One lime juice
- Three tbsp of vegan mayo
- A roughly chopped small gem lettuce
- A can of kidney beans
- Three tbsp of jerk seasoning
- A tin of rinsed and drained young jackfruit
- A large peeled and wedged sweet potato

Method

Preheat oven to 350F

Mix in some pepper, salt and some olive oil with the sweet potatoes and toss them.

Bake the potatoes in the oven, in a baking tray for twenty minutes. Halfway check and turn them to cook evenly.

Season the rinsed jackfruit with two tsp of jerk seasoning.

In a pan over low heat cook the jackfruit in a tbsp of olive oil for five minutes stirring ad it cooks. Ensure the jackfruit is well softened before you remove it from the heat. When well cooked, shred it using two forks.

Stir in the cooked jackfruit with the kidney beans over medium heat for another few minutes.

Taste the food and if need be, add more of the seasoning.

In a bowl, mix the pepper, lime juice, and mayo. Taste and balance the ingredients where necessary.

Start the wrapping process by including a bit of each. Put lettuce, a sixth off the jackfruit mixture, some potato wedges and a pleasant touch of the mayo mixture. Wrap up the food.

You can eat it right away, and it can last a couple of days in the fridge.

Jackfruit tacos

Ingredients

- Vegan blue cheese
- Two tbsp of chopped chives
- A cupful of sliced white cabbage

- A cupful of sliced red cabbage
- Three quarter cups of buffalo sauce
- A can of jackfruit
- Six taco shells

Method

Bring the drained jackfruit to boil in three cups of water over medium heat in a pan. Let the jackfruit boil for five minutes.

When softened, drain off for the water and tear it down with a pair of forks. Put it in a pan and pour it in the buffalo sauce. Let the food cook over medium heat for seven minutes. The jackfruit turns dark. Turn down the heat when cooked. For the tacos, dress with avocado and cabbage mix and put toppings of the chives and the blue cheese.

Jackfruit tacos with garlic sauce

Ingredients for the filling

- A tsp of cumin
- A tbsp of chili powder
- 14.5 Oz can have diced tomatoes
- A minced garlic cloves
- Half cup of diced red onions
- A can of green jackfruit

Ingredients for the white garlic sauce

- An eighth tsp of salt
- Half cup of almond milk

- A tsp of cumin
- Two tbsp of nutritional yeast
- Two garlic cloves
- A quarter cup of soaked raw cashews

Ingredients for serving

Topping; shredded cabbage, hot other sauce, diced tomatoes, and sliced peppers.

86" tortilla shells

Method for preparing the filling

Drain the jackfruit and rinse it. Do away with the two tips. Tear the jackfruit into pieces.

In two tsp of water, Water the minced garlic and onions chop over medium heat. Include the shredded jackfruit along with the other components. Once they boil, simmer and let the food cook for ten minutes while covered.

Method for making the garlic sauce

Strain off the water from the cashews. Blend all the sauce ingredients in a food processor or till they smoothen. The process should take half an hour.

Bring together the components. Fill the tortillas and top them with the toppings. Sprinkle on with the garlic sauce.

Jackfruit pie

Filling Ingredients

- Half cup frozen peas
- Three-quarter cups of ringed carrots
- Three-quarter cups of diced potatoes
- A tbsp of olive oil
- Two rosemary sprigs
- Two bay leaves
- Two pressed garlic cloves
- Half diced yellow onion
- Two half cups of unsweetened almond milk
- A can of green jackfruit

Roux Ingredients

- A half-pint of almond milk
- Three tbsp of vegan butter
- Three tbsp of plain flour

Pastry Ingredients

- A tsp of melted vegan butter
- Two Oz of vegan puff pastry

Method

Rinse the jackfruit off and remove the inner core.

Fry the jackfruit in the onions and olive on a pan over medium heat for at least three minutes till the onions brown. Include two cups of almond milk, the rosemary, bay leaves, and garlic. Stir the mixture, place on a lid and lower the heat.

It should cook for at least twenty-five minutes for the jackfruit to soften. When softened use forks to bring it apart. Stir and include the remaining half cup of almond milk. Put in the peas, potatoes and carrots. Turn up the heat to cook on medium for a few minutes and reduce to a simmer.

When cooked, remove the rosemary and bay leaves for the food and throw them away. Turn down the heat and strain off the excess liquid from the food.

To the strained liquid, add more almond milk to make half a pint.

On a clean pan, heat the butter to melt under medium heat and then put in the flour. Whisk the mixture to form a paste and let it cook for two minutes. Pour in half of the almond milk to the mixture. Whisk the dough and let it cook till it starts to thicken. Once the mixture gains consistency, include the remaining almond milk and mix well. Turn off the heat and mix in the vegetables.

Put the mixture in a casserole. Pour out the pastry on a floured flat surface and roll it into a flat seven-inch thick disk. Lay it over the pan and use a fork to apply pressure on the sides. Do two slits on it.

Preheat the oven to 375F and cook the pastry in it for twenty minutes. The top should come off brownish.

Sticky barbecue rib

Ingredients

- Four tbs of barbecue sauce
- Two tbs of low salt soy sauce
- A tsp of black pepper
- A tsp of garlic powder
- Two tsp of onion powder
- A tbsp of smoked paprika
- Two tbsp of nutritional yeast
- Seven oz of vegetable stock
- Five oz of vita wheat gluten

Method

Preheat fan oven to 356F

Combine black pepper, garlic, onions, smoked paprika, nutritional yeast and the heat gluten in a bowl. Stir the mixture. Include the soy sauce and vegetable stock and combine. You can add more gluten to make the dough less sticky. Knead the dough.

Line a foil a baking tray and lay the dough in a one-centimeter thin layer. Make it in the form of a rack of ribs. Cook it in the oven for twenty minutes till it assumes a golden appearance. Halfway, turn it took evenly on both sides.

When well done, remove from the oven. Sprinkle two teaspoons of barbecue sauce on both sides.

Pour some little oil in a frying pan and heat over medium heat. Cook the seitan in the pan for a few minutes and turn on either side to assume a crispy feel.

Enjoy while warm!

Beet mushrooms and black been burger

Ingredients

- Salt
- Half tbsp of cumin
- A tbsp of soy sauce
- A tbsp of cayenne
- A quarter block tofu of 15oz
- A quarter cup of quick cook oats
- Half chopped yellow onion
- Eight oz of mushroom
- A large diced beet
- Two cups of cooked black beans

Method

Preheat your oven to 400F.

Toss the finely diced beets in olive oil and roast them to soften for half an hour.

Cut the mushrooms into dices, sprinkle on some olive oil and fry under medium heat to dehydrate.

Put the remaining ingredients in a food processor and blend to make some uneven dough.

Oil a baking sheet. Form six parties of the mixture and place them on the baking sheet. Cook in the preheated oven for twenty minutes. Turn after ten minutes of baking to cook evenly on both sides.

Lime tart

Base ingredients

- A pinch of sea salt
- Half teaspoon of grated ginger
- Half tsp of vanilla extract
- A tbsp of coconut oil
- Three-quarter cups of desiccated coconut
- A cupful of dates
- A cupful of almonds

Filling ingredients include

- A pinch of sea salt
- A tbsp of lime zest
- One-third cup of coconut nectar
- Three-quarter cups of softened and chilled coconut oil
- A cup of like segments
- Two cups of ripe avocado

Topping ingredients

- Extra zest for garnishing
- Half cup of cashews

- Three-quarter cups of coconut cream

Method

Blend all the basing ingredients. They should give a breadcrumb-like appearance but sticky.

Line up a tart tin with clear wrap and our out the blended mixture inside. Spread the mixture evenly in and up the tin. Put it in the freezer and move on to work on the other ingredients.

In a high-speed processor, process all the filling ingredients to a smooth pulp. The mixture should come off free of lumps and avocado aroma. Take the base out of the freezer and fill in up with the processed mixture. Smoothen the top part and place it back in the fridge overnight.

For the toppings, blend the cashews and coconut cream. Serve the cream with the tart separately. Alternatively, dollop the cream in the middle of the tart.

Lentil meat balls with pasta

Ingredients for meatballs

- Deep frying oil
- Half cup of breadcrumbs
- Half tsp of salt
- Half tsp of coriander powder
- Half tsp of cumin powder
- Two garlic cloves
- An onion

- A cup of whole red lentils

Ingredients for pasta

- Four tbsp of vegan parmesan cheese
- Four basil leaves
- One and a half tsp of red chili flakes
- One tbsp of parsley
- A tbsp of oregano
- Four garlic cloves
- Salt
- A tbsp of olive oil
- A packet of pasta

Method

Clean up the lentils and soak them in water for half an hour. Remove them and put them in a pressure cooker with little water. Cook them to soften.

Grate the beets free of the skin. Slice the garlic and onions to small pieces.

Mix the salt, coriander powder, cumin powder, garlic powder, chopped onions, lentil paste and grated beets in a bowl.

In a frying pan, heat the oil. Use your hands to form small sized balls of the mixture and deep fry them to golden brownish color. When cooked, drain them in a kitchen paper.

Follow the manufacturer's instructions in cooking the pasta. When the pasta is well done, drain them and run cold water in them and drain it immediately. Put in a tsp of olive oil and toss them in the oil.

Fry the garlic in olive oil in a pan. Include salt, chili flakes and the herbs to the cooked garlic. Include the pasta in this fried formula and toss. Immediately serve the pasta in plates. Include the cooked meat balls and top it with vegan parmesan cheese.

Chapter 4:

Seasonal Recipes

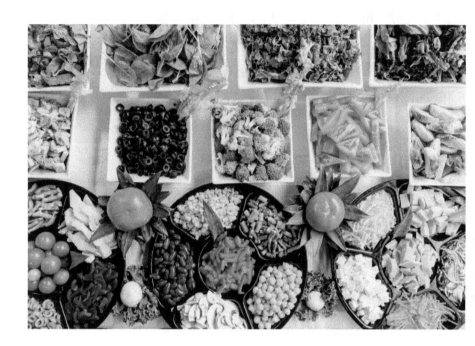

Recipes for the spring season

Chocolate cherry cookies

Ingredients

- Three tsp of morello cherry juice
- Half cup of no vanilla milk
- A cupful of semi-sweet chocolate chips
- Two dozen of morello cherries in syrup
- A quarter tsp of baking soda
- A quarter tsp of baking powder

- A quarter tsp of sea salt
- Half cup of unsweetened cocoa powder
- One and a half cups of all-purpose flour
- One and a half tsp of vanilla extract
- Mashed half ripe banana
- A cup of sugar
- Half cup of vegan butter

Method

Preheat oven to 350F

Combine the sugar and butter in medium speed in a mixing bowl. Mix in the vanilla and mashed banana.

In a different bowl, put in the baking soda, baking powder, salt, cocoa, and all-purpose flour and mix.

Put together both mixtures in the blender and combine under medium speed to give a thick batter.

Place the batter on the baking pan in equal scoops and press a finger lightly in the middle of each. On the print formed, place a cherry. Do the same for all the cookies.

Mix the none dairy milk with the chocolate chips in a pot and cook over medium heat stir the mixture till it's all melted. Turn off the heat and pour in the cherry juice to the melted mixture. On each cookie, place a tsp of the mixture.

Let the cookies cook in the oven for about ten minutes. When done remove from the oven and give them time to cool down before placing another spoonful of the chocolate mixture on the same spot as the previous.

Mozzarella quinoa meatballs

Ingredients

- Fresh parsley for garnishing
- Marinara sauce
- A cup of chopped and grated vegan mozzarella
- A tsp of lemon zest
- Half tsp of salt
- A tsp of paprika
- A tsp of dried oregano
- A tsp of dried basil
- Two minced garlic cloves
- A finely diced yellow onion
- Two tbsp of olive oil
- Three tbsp of water
- A tbsp of flax meal
- A cup of rinsed and drained quinoa

Method

Prepare the quinoa as per the manufacturer's instructions

Mix flaxseed meal with water in a bowl and place aside.

Sauté the onions with a tbsp of olive oil in a pan. Add salt, paprika, dried oregano, dried basil and garlic. Include the quinoa and mix. When the ingredients are well cooked set aside in a bowl. Mix in the cheese shreds, lemon zest, and flaxseed. Form a dozen even balls of the mixture and keep refrigerated for half an hour.

Preheat your oven to 400F. Apply the remaining olive oil on the balls and let them cook in the oven for twenty minutes.

Ready to serve when cooked. They should attain a brown color. When serving, top the meatballs with parsley and marinara sauce.

A grilled Cheese sandwich and blackberry lemon lavender

Ingredients

- Macadamia ricotta
- Vegan butter
- Eight slices of bread
- A quarter tsp of salt
- Half tsp of lemon zest
- A tsp of dried lavender
- A tbsp of arrow root powder or corn starch
- A tbsp of agave syrup
- A tbsp of fresh lemon juice
- A tsps. of water
- Two cups of frozen or fresh or blackberries

Method

In a cooking pot, boil the mixture of salt, lemon zest, lavender, arrow root powder\corn starch, agave syrup, lemon juice and water over high heat and reduce to low and simmer. Ensure the mixture is still boiling when simmered. Stir the food as you cook. It should cook till it thickens and should take for six minutes.

Bring out two slices of the bread. On the outer part of the slices apply the vegan butter. On the inner part of one slice apply the blackberry sauce and on the other slice, apply macadamia ricotta. Combine the two slices and use the same procedure to do remaining three pairs.

Cook the slices in a large frying pan over medium heat. You can place several of the sandwiches at a time. Once one side turns golden brown turn over and cooks the other side, serve the sandwiches while they are still hot.

If the sauce is left over, keep refrigerated in a closed container for a maximum of five days.

Lemon strawberry scones with lemon glaze

Ingredients

- Lemon glaze components
- A tbsp of fresh lemon juice
- Half cup of sugar or xylitol

Dry ingredients

- Two tsp of lemon zest
- Half tsp of salt
- Half tsp of baking soda
- A tbsp of baking powder
- Half cup of coconut sugar

- One and a quarter cups of oat flour
- One and a half cups of spelled flour

Wet ingredients

- Five tbsp of chilled vegan butter
- A tsp of vanilla extract
- Two tsp of fresh lemon juice
- Half cup of almond milk
- *Add-ins;* a cupful of strawberry dices

Method of preparation

Line a preheated oven at 425F with a baking sheet and parchment paper.

Combine the lemon juice and almond milk in a cup and leave it aside.

Pour out all the dry ingredients in a bowl and mix thoroughly.

Break the butter to pea-sized pieces.

To the lemon-almond milk mixture, add the lemon zest and vanilla extract. Add the wet mixture onto the dry ingredients and slightly combine without overdoing it. The strawberries should go into the sticky dough so gently fold them in.

Place the dough on to a floured flat surface. Flour your hands to prevent it from sticking. Sprinkle some flour on the dough because it will turn out too sticky. Press on it to form a twelve-inch disc. Split the flour into triangular shapes with the help of a sharp knife. Gently pick up the sliced pieces and place them on the baking sheet.

Place them in the oven and bake to a golden color which will take between seventeen and fifteen minutes. When cooked, move them to a cooling rack.

Combine the glazing ingredients and drizzle them on the cooled scones.

They are now ready to serve.

Blueberry Lemon granola

Wet Ingredients

- Up to 15 drops of plain stevia
- One lemon zest
- A tsp of melted coconut oil
- Half cup of fresh lemon juice
- Half cup of brown rice syrup

Dry Ingredients

- Two tsp of ground cinnamon
- Half cup of hemp seeds
- One and a half cups of dried blueberries
- Two cups of gluten-free rolled oats
- Three cups of puffed millet
- Three cups of plain corn flakes

Method

Line your 275F preheated oven with baking two sheets with parchment paper.

Combine the dry and wet components in different bowls. Once well combined, pour the wet ingredients onto the dry mixture. Share out the combined mixture evenly between the two baking sheets.

Cook the two sheets alternatively in the oven to allow even cooking. Interchanging the shelves, they are cooking at. Bake for forty-five minutes and remove from the oven. When sufficiently cooled, you can store it in an air tight container.

Mung beans

Ingredients

- A tbsp of olive oil
- Two tbsp of arrow root
- Two thirds cup of almond or soy milk
- Three tbsp nutritional yeast
- Two tbsp of tamari or soy sauce
- Half tbsp of turmeric
- Two tsp of Dijon mustard
- A pack of firm tofu
- A handful of fresh basil leaves
- 100grams of baby spinach
- 100grams of chopped kale
- Three chopped mushrooms
- Four crushed and chopped garlic
- Four chopped spring onions
- Half chopped onion
- One chopped yellow pepper

- An egg substitute such as flax

Method

Mix the cooked rice with the flax or egg replacer and pour it in to a spring pan. Brush on some oil on top of the mixture in the pan and Cook it in an oven at 375F. Let it cook for ten minutes.

Cook the white scallions or spring onions along with the regular onion chopping in a frying pan with oil. When softened include mushrooms and pepper and cook under medium heat for ten minutes.

Include the green scallions, basil, spinach, kales, and spinach. Mix them in and cook to wilt then lower the heat to a simmer.

In a blender or food processor include the oil, arrowroot, milk, nutritional yeast, soy sauce, tofu, and turmeric and blend them to smooth paste.

Combine the blended mixture with the greens. Stir in the tofu mixture till well combined. Add the mixture on to the baked rice.

Preheat the oven to 350F and place the mixture inside. Cook for forty-five minutes. However, keep checking to make sure it doesn't burn. Remove the food when it starts to brown. Let the food sit for 60minutes before removing the hard-outer part. Slice it when fully cooled.

It can be eaten alongside a salad for any meal of the day.

Cacao berry bowl

Ingredients

- A tsp of hemp hearts
- Two teaspoons of cacao nibs
- Half cup of mixed raspberries, blue berries, and blackberries.
- Three thinly sliced strawberries
- Half thinly sliced a ripe banana
- Half and a quarter cup of separate cacao quinoa granola
- Two-tab spoons of cacao powder
- A tsp of maca powder
- A packet of acai powder
- One and quarter cup of frozen mixed berries
- Half ripe banana
- Half cup pf vegan milk or almond milk

Method

Place the serving bowl in the freezer to help in keeping the food cold.

Slice the half banana and strawberry and for the topping and place in separate bowls

Blend the milk, half-ripe banana, frozen berries, the acai powder, and maca powder in a high-speed blender to smoothen. Scrape off the sides of the blender as you blend and stir to break up the lumps that form.

Get your bowl out of the fridge and place the quarter cup of granola inside. Include the blended mixture in the bowl. Place the other half cup granolas on top.

Pace the sliced fruits on top then sprinkle on the hemp seeds and cacao nibs on the mixture.

Refrigerate it to chill before serving.

Carrot lox

Ingredients

- Half rap of coconut vinegar
- Two tsp of liquid smoke
- A table spoon of olive oil
- Three large unpeeled carrots
- Two cups of course sea salt

Serving ingredients

- Fresh dill minced red onions
- Capers
- Vegan cream cheese
- Bagels

Method

Preheat the oven to 375F

Put the cleaned and unpeeled carrots in a glass Pyrex that fits them while still wet. Fill in with the coarse salt. Don't let the carrots touch the glass surface. Let the carrots cook in the oven for 90minutes.

When cooked, remove from the oven and pour them out onto a flat surface. Let them cool slightly and scape off the salt. Peel off any skin remains and chop the carrots into thin, jagged strips.

Mix the coconut vinegar, liquid smoke, and olive oil and whisk them thoroughly. Use the mixture to marinate the carrots. Make sure they are well covered in the mixture. Add more olive oil to make them softer if need be.

Place the carrots in the refrigerator for 48hrs to allow the flavor to sink in and for the carrots to soften and assume a silky texture.

When serving, take the carrots out of the refrigerator and allow enough time for them to attain room temperature.

Put together fresh sprigs of dill, red onions, vegan cream cheese, capers, and a toasted bagel. Or otherwise, as you desire.

Carrot cake granola

Ingredients

- The dry ingredients
- Half tsp of cloves
- three quarter teaspoons of nutmeg
- A tsp of ground ginger
- Two and a half tsp of cinnamon
- A three-quarter cup of raisins
- A cupful of chopped pecans
- A cupful of flax meal
- Four cups of rolled oats

Wet ingredients

- One quarter cup and separate one eight cups of agave syrup

- One quarter cup and different one eighth cup of molasses
- Half cup of canola oil
- Three quarter cups of Apple juice
- Three-quarter cups of finely grated carrots

Method of preparation

Preheat your oven to 275F

Line it with two baking sheets with parchment paper

Apply the vegan spray to prevent the food from sticking

Leave aside the grated carrots and combine the wet ingredients separately from the dry one. Place the wet ingredients in the microwave and let them heat for a minute. When hot, mix in the grated carrots.

Include the wet mixture on to the dry components and combine them well. Divide the mixture between the two baking sheets and spread them evenly on the surface. Make some numerous small clusters on the mixture by use of your hands.

Place the taking sheets one in the lower oven compartment and the other in the upper one. After twenty-five minutes, interchange the baking sheets to allow them to cook evenly. After interchanging, bake the food for twenty minutes. Let it cool down before removing from the sheets. When sufficiently cooled place in a container and tightly close it.

Peach green tea smoothie

Ingredients

- A tbsp of matcha powder
- A tsp of maca powder
- A tbsp of buckwheat groats
- A tbsp of hemp seeds
- One and a half cup of frozen peach slices
- One and a half cup of frozen mango slices or if you prefer to use banana
- Two handfuls of leafy greens
- A cup of almond milk

Method

Include all the components in a blender and blend till they smoothen. It is ready to drink. You can use the topping of your choice for this smoothie.

Baked tofu and cauliflower

Ingredients for making the tofu

- A quarter cup of fresh lemon juice
- Ten ounces of firm tofu. Divided into quarters packed in an air free package.
- A tbs of low sodium tamari
- A tbsp pf extra Virgin olive oil

Ingredients for making the benedict

- Chopped parsley for garnishing
- One sliced tomato
- Two English muffins halved

Ingredients for making the cauliflower hollandaise

- Freshly ground pepper
- Salt
- An eight of a tsp turmeric
- A quarter tsp of chili powder
- Two tsp of white miso paste
- A cupful of great northern beans
- Two tbsp of fresh lemon juice
- Two tbsp of nutritional yeast flakes
- A cup of non dairy milk
- A minced garlic clove
- Three quarter cups of diced yellow onions
- Two separate rooms of virgin olive oil
- A half cauliflower

Method

Preheat oven to 425F

Line in with baking sheet with parchment. On the baking sheet, line the cauliflower florets tossed in olive oil. Let the florets bake in the oven for twenty minutes. Halfway baking toss them to allow even cooking.

As the cauliflower is roasting, fry the garlic and onions in a teaspoon of olive oil on a skillet and medium heat. Cook for six minutes till they look translucent, fragrant and soft. You can lower the heat for them to cook without sticking to the pan.

In a high-speed blender, put together the remaining ingredients, the cooed onions, and the roasted cauliflower.

Procedure for preparing the tofu

Preheat the oven to 400F. Line an 8 by 8 baking sheet. Put together the tamari and extra virgin olive oil. Coat the tofu slices in the tamari mixture. Cook in the oven for 20mins. Turn over the tofu and include lemon juice in the pan. Place back the baking sheet to the oven and let it cook for another 20mins.

Procedure for making the benedict

In a toaster, toast the slices of English muffins. Top the toasted slices with tomato slices and a tofu slice. Place the hollandaise sauce on top and the parsley chops.

Ready to serve.

Carrot cake waffles with cinnamon maple cream cheese

Ingredients

Cinnamon maple cheese ingredients

- Half tsp of vanilla extract
- A tsp of cinnamon

- A tsp of fresh lemon juice
- Two tsp of maple syrup
- Half cup of vegan cream cheese

Wet ingredients

- A cupful of finely grated carrots
- A tsp of vanilla extract
- A tsp of fresh lemon juice
- Two tbsp. of maple syrup
- Two tbsp. of melted coconut oil
- Two thirds cup of almond milk
- One and a half cups of plain soy or coconut yoghurt

Dry ingredients

- Half tsp of nutmeg
- A tsp of cloves
- A tsp of cinnamon
- Two tsp of baking powder
- Half tsp of salt
- Half cup of sorghum flour
- Half cup of brown rice flour
- A cupful of oat flour

Add-ins include two thirds cup of raisins and make sure you have excess for topping.

Method

Whip together the maple syrup, cinnamon, and the cream cheese till fluffy. Put the whipped mixture in the fridge as you work on the other ingredients.

Mix the dry ingredients in a bowl.

In a separate bowl, put together the wet ingredients as listed above and combine them. Pour the wet mixture on to the dry and combine the two without overdoing it. In the mixture, fold in the raisins and carrots and leave the dough for at least ten minutes. In the meantime, heat the waffle maker. Make the waffles depending on the type of machine you are using. Use the cinnamon maple cream cheese sauce you made to top up and maple syrup. Enjoy while warm.

Dragon fruit smoothie

Ingredients for the smoothie

- Half scoop of vegan protein smoothie powder
- Half cup of almond milk
- Half peeled kiwifruit
- Two handfuls of baby spinach
- A packet of frozen pitaya
- A cupful of chopped frozen pineapples
- A cupful of frozen chopped mangoes

Ingredients for making the bowl

Chopped fruits; raspberries, blackberries, blueberries, mango, kiwifruit, banana, and strawberries

The granola of your choice

Method

Put all the smoothie making ingredients listed above in a blender and blend to a smooth paste.

Add a quarter cup of the granola into the serving bowl. Pour in the smoothies on top of the granola. Add more granola toppings to the bowl and the fruit slices of choice. Enjoy the smoothie immediately.

Peach and cream doughnuts

Wet ingredients

- A tsp of vanilla extract
- A tbsp. of melted butter
- A tsp of apple cedar vinegar
- Three quarter cup of almond milk

The dry ingredients

- Half tsp of salt
- A quarter tsp of cinnamon
- A tsp of baking powder
- One and a half tsp of egg replacer
- A cupful of wheat pastry flour

Additional ingredients

- Three tbsp. of almond milk
- Half tsp of vanilla extract
- Half cup of sugar or xylitol

- Two small peaches or one large peach

Method

Preheat your oven to 350F

Grease a doughnut pan.

Pour together the apple cedar vinegar and the almond milk and let it sit for ten minutes before using it.

Whisk the dry ingredients together in a larger bowl. In a smaller bowl mix in the wet ingredients and include the almond milk vinegar mixture. Pour in the wet mixture to the dry one and combine without overdoing it.

In the wells of the doughnut pan spread the peach pieces. Use a pastry bag to squeeze the dough into the doughnut pan covering the peach pieces. As you press in the dough, leave one third of the well unfilled.

Cook the doughnuts in the preheated oven for about ten minutes till they assume the golden doughnut color. When well cooked, remove from the oven and give them time to cool down before placing them on the cooling rack.

As the doughnuts cool, in a bowl, mix the half tsp of vanilla extract and sugar or xylitol. Pour in the almond milk as you stir till you achieve your desired consistence. Dip the cooled doughnut top part into this mixture.

You can also drizzle the mixture on the doughnuts and top it with pistachio pieces.

Soy free vegan benedict

Ingredients for hollandaise sauce

- Salt to taste
- A quarter tsp of garlic powder
- A quarter tsp of onion powder
- Half tsp of turmeric
- Half tsp of Dijon mustard
- Two tbsp. of nutritional yeast
- Juice of one lemon
- Extra water for soaking cashew
- A cupful of soaked cashews

Ingredients for the chickpea patties

- Olive oil spray
- Two tbsp. of olive oil
- A quarter tsp of turmeric
- A quarter tsp of smoked paprika
- Threes quarter tsps. of garlic powder
- Three quarter tsp of onion powder
- A tbsp. of black salt
- Two cups of chickpea flour
- Four cups of water

Assembling ingredients

- Eight asparagus spears

- One thinly sliced large tomato

- A shiitake bacon

- Two English muffins

Method for preparing the chickpea patties

Put together the spices, salt and chickpea flour in a bowl and mix.

Line a baking sheet with parchment paper

Boil the water in a cooking pot. As it boils, stir in the chickpea flour as it boils. Let the mixture attain consistency.

Add the olive oil to the mixture and stir in for a minute. Turn down the heat and pour out the mixture into the lined baking tin. Refrigerate the mixture for ten hours while el covered.

Remove the mixture from the refrigerator when ready to cook. Lift the refrigerated mixture out by holding on to the parchment paper. Have it on a flat board and cut out the mixture into four round patties using a biscuit or cookie cutter. The remains of the dough can be used as sandwich fillers when baked for around twenty minutes in the lined baking pan.

Over medium heat, heat up a nonstick pan. Spray on with the olive oil and fry the patties for four minutes. When they brown on the part in contact with the pan, flip and cook the other side while the pan is covered for four minutes. Remove the patties when they are crispy and golden. Place them on kitchen paper when cooked and repeat the same process till all the patties are done.

Bake both the patties and cut outs in the oven for twenty minutes at 400F. Halfway baking, flip them to cook evenly on both sides. They should come off firm and brownish all round. Take them out of the oven when well cooked.

Method for preparing the hollandaise sauce

Drain off the cashews without discarding the water. Set the cashew water aside. With thirteen teaspoons of water, blend the hollandaise sauce ingredients in the processor till smooth. Pour it into a bowl and chill.

Assembling method

Steam the asparagus. To do this, you could use a steaming pot. Steam the asparagus for seven minutes and set it aside.

Split the English muffins and toast them.

Place the shiitake bacon on each of the toasted muffins. On the bacon, place the chickpea patty. Top it with a tomato slice and the asparagus spears. Finally, pour on the hollandaise sauce. You can split the benedict into halves or just have it whole.

Find the recipe for the shiitake bacon below.

Shiitake bacon

Ingredients

- Two cups of thinly sliced shiitake mushroom caps
- Half cup of smoked paprika
- One tsp of sesame oil
- Three quarter tsp of liquid smoke
- A quarter tsp of salt

- One tbsp. of olive oil

Method for preparation

Preheat oven to 350F

Include all the ingredients in a bowl and combine. You can whisk them to combine properly.

Include the shitake mushroom and mix. Let the mushroom to take in the flavors for about sixty minutes. Over a baking sheet, place on a silpat. Place a thin layer of the mushrooms on the silpat. Cook the mushrooms in the oven for ten minutes. After ten minutes, turn the mushrooms to cook evenly on both sides. Cook for another fifteen minutes. Turn the oven to 375F and bake for an additional ten minutes. Turn the mushrooms once more and cook for another ten minutes. If the food starts to burn remove them from the oven. Drain the oil in paper towels. Eat while still warm.

Lemon muffins

Ingredients

- Half cup of almond meal
- Half cup of rolled oats
- A cupful of whole heat pastry flour
- A tbsp. of poppy seeds
- One and a half cup of baking soda
- Half tsp of sea salt
- A one third cup of natural cane sugar
- A quarter cup of agave nectar or maple syrup

- A quarter cup of unsweetened almond milk
- A quarter cup of melted avocado oil or coconut oil
- A tsp of lemon juice or vanilla extract
- One third cup of Meyer lemon juice
- Two tbsp. of Meyer lemon zest
- Three quarter cups of unsweetened apple sauce
- Two batches of flex eggs

Ingredients for the glaze

- A tbsp. of lemon juice
- A cupful of powdered sugar

Method

Set the flax egg in a bowl and leave it for five minutes. Line a baking tin for twelve muffins with liners. Preheat oven to 375.

Whisk salt, baking soda, cane sugar, agave or maple syrup, almond milk, oil, lemon juice, lemon zest, and apple sauce. Expect the mixture to foam from the baking soda-lemon juice reaction. Include the oats, almond meal, and flour and mix without overdoing it. Include the poppy seeds into the mixture.

Scoop the dough into the muffin tins evenly. Bake in the oven for half an hour and check to see if well done.

Once cooked, let it sit in the baking tin for five minutes to cook before transferring the muffins into a cooling rack. Pour the lemon juice and sugar powder into a bowl and whisk. Drizzle the whisked mixture over the cooked muffins.

You can freeze the muffins and have them edible for up to one month. All the same, you can eat them for up to seven days when well covered even at room temperature.

Rainbow kelp noodle salad and ginger almond lemon dressing

Ingredients for the salad

- Sesame seeds
- Chopped almonds
- Two cups of chopped mango
- A quarter cup of chopped cilantro
- Three cups of baby spinach
- A quarter head of thinly sliced red cabbage
- One thinly sliced bell pepper
- Two julienned carrots
- A package of rinsed kelp noodles

Ingredients for the salad dressing

- Half tsp of white miso
- A tsp of tamari /soy sauce or liquid aminos
- A tsp of ground ginger
- A tbsp. of agave syrup
- Two tbsp. of apple cedar vinegar
- A quarter cup of lemon juice
- Half cup of water for soaking

Method

Blend all the dressing ingredients as listed, in a food processor or blend till smooth.

In a separate bowl, put together the cilantro, red cabbage, bell pepper, carrots, spinach, and the kelp noodles, and mix.

Combine with the blended dressing and toss till evenly mixed. You can top the salad with sesame seeds, chopped almonds, and mango.

Quinoa salad with avocado, peas, asparagus and basil lemon dressing

Ingredients for the salad

- A quarter cup of chopped basil
- Freshly ground black pepper
- Salt
- A chopped avocado
- A cupful of frozen peas
- A tbsp. of fresh lemon juice
- A bunch of asparagus
- Two tsp of olive oil
- Half tsp of salt
- A cupful of quinoa
- Two cups of water

Ingredients for dressing

- Freshly ground black pepper

- Salt
- A tbsp. of finely chopped basil
- A minced garlic clove
- A tsp of agave nectar or honey
- Three tbsp. of fresh lemon juice
- Three tbsp. of olive oil

Method

Mix the dressing ingredients in a bowl by whisking and keep aside.

In a saucepan boil the quinoa in some water over medium heat for five minutes. Lower the heat to a simmer while still boiling and cook until all the water is fully absorbed. When dry turn off the heat and fluff using a fork.

Over medium heat in a skillet, heat the olive oil and cook in the asparagus with the lemon juice till soft. The cooking should take five minutes. When the asparagus is well done, add the peas and cook for another two minutes then turn off the heat.

In a separate clean bowl, include the avocado, peas and asparagus, and the quinoa. Combine the mixture till evenly distributed and then add the dressing. Make sure the dressing is evenly mixed in the salad. Add some pepper and salt to your liking and then add the fresh chopped basil. Mix in the basil and serve the salad while still fresh.

Citrus basil salad with balsamic jam dressing

Ingredients

- One quarter cup of water

- A tsp of balsamic vinegar
- A tbsp. of cherry jam
- A quarter cup of fresh basil
- Two blood oranges
- Two grapefruits
- Four oranges of different varieties

Method

Chop the peeled citrus fruits in even rounded slices and put them together in a bowl.

Chop the basil and toss them together.

Whisk the water, vinegar, and jam in a bowl. Use this mixture to dress your fruit salad. There will be left over you can use later if refrigerated.

Chicken free cabbage salad

Ingredients for the dressing

- A tsp of sesame seeds
- A tsp of Dijon mustard
- Half tbsp. of maple syrup
- Half tbsp. of tahini
- One eighth of a cup of apple cedar vinegar
- A quarter cup of orange juice

Salad ingredients

- Sesame seeds for garnishing

- Pepper and salt to taste
- Olive oil spray
- A handful of string beans
- Four finely chopped green onions
- Three large carrots
- One nectarine cut in half, pitted and sliced
- Half cabbage head that has been quartered and shredded

Ingredients for preparing the tofu

- Half tsp of liquid smoke
- Half tsp of paprika
- Half tsp of onion powder
- Half tsp of garlic powder
- Half tsp of marjoram a tsp of dried thyme
- A quarter cup of brag liquid aminos
- Half cup of vegetable broth
- A pressed block of tofu

Method

In a shallow container, put together the tofu marinade ingredients.

Split the tofu slices into two and break it further into smaller pieces. Place the pieces on the marinade mixture and refrigerate for half an hour. After fifteen minutes, flip the tofu to marinate evenly on both sides.

When done, preheat your oven to 350F. Take a baking sheet and line it up with parchment paper on. Use olive oil spray to grease.

Drain off the excess marinade and bake in the oven on the already prepared baking sheet for half an hour. Halfway baking flip the tofu to cook evenly on all sides. When well cooked, take it out of the oven and keep aside.

In a baking sheet, place your string of beans and toss them in olive oil salt and pepper. Turn your oven to 400F and bake in the beans for up to ten minutes. Halfway baking flip the beans to roast evenly.

Start on the salad. For the dressing, include all the ingredients (setting aside the sesame seeds) in an immersion blender and blend to a smooth mixture. Include the sesame seeds and lightly blend them by pulsing twice. Chill the mixture.

Put together the green onions, carrots, avocado, nectarine, and cabbage in a bowl and combine them. Include the cooled tofu and bean strings. Add the dressing then toss the mixture till evenly combined. Sprinkle on the sesame seeds for garnishing and enjoy the salad immediately.

Caesar salad

Ingredients for preparing the lettuce

- Ten cups of chopped romaine lettuce (to small heads)
- Five cups of chopped Lacinato kale (a small bunch)

Ingredients for the nut and seeds parmesan cheese

- Finely grained seas salt
- Half tsp of garlic powder
- A tbsp. of extra virgin olive oil

- A tbsp. of nutritional yeast
- A small garlic clove
- Two tbsp. of hulled hemp seeds
- One third cup of raw cashews

Dressing ingredients

- Pepper
- Half tsp of fine grain sea salt
- Two tsp of capers
- Half tbsp. of vegan Worcestershire sauce
- A small garlic clove
- Half tbsp. of Dijon mustard
- A tbsp. of lemon juice
- Two tbsp. of extra virgin olive oil
- A quarter cup of water
- Half cup of pre-soaked cashews

Roasted chickpea croutons ingredients

- A quarter tsp of cayenne pepper
- Half tsp of garlic powder
- Half tsp of fine grain sea salt
- A tsp of extra virgin olive oil
- One and a half cups of cooked chickpeas/ a can of drained and rinsed chickpeas

Method

Pre-soak the cashews over-night. Make sure the pre-soaked cashews are drained and well rinsed before use.

In case you are using canned chickpeas, drain them and rinse thoroughly. Dry off the water and moisture by rubbing on a clean kitchen towel. Place them in a baking sheet and sprinkle on with olive oil. Add cayenne, salt and garlic powder and toss them till evenly seasoned.

Preheat your oven to 400F and roast in the chickpeas for twenty minutes. Turn the chickpeas by gently rolling them in the baking sheet and then return them in the oven to cook for another twenty minutes till they assume a golden coating.

As for the dressing, include all the dressing ingredients leaving aside the salt into a high-speed blender. Put in the cashews and blend to a smooth paste. If need be, add some water in the mixture if you are experiencing difficulties in getting them done. Mix in the salt and taste to adjust.

In preparing the cheese, include the garlic and cashews in a food processor and chop till finely processed. Include the remaining cheese ingredients and pulse till evenly mixed. Include the salt and mix it in the blended ingredients.

In preparing the lettuce, remove the kales from the stems and chop them finely. Use a salad spinner to dry the chopped kales then transfer them into a larger bowl. Cut the romaine into medium sized pieces and wash them. Dry the chopped romaine in the salad spinner too. Include the dried romaine chops together with the kales. The mixture should make up to 15 cups.

Pour the dressing on the lettuce and mix by tossing the mixture. Add a pinch of salt and combine. Add the parmesan cheese and the roasted chickpeas by sprinkling them on the mixture. Serve immediately.

Almond carrot soup with skillet roasted chickpeas

Ingredients

- Skillet roasted chickpeas
- Pepper and salt to taste
- A tbsp. of maple syrup
- Two tbsp. of fresh lime juice
- Three tbsp. of sriracha sauce
- 2/3cups of creamy almond butter
- Two cups of water
- Four cups of vegetable broth
- Half tsp of ground ginger
- Half tsp of smoked paprika
- A tsp of ancho chili powder
- A tsp of ground coriander
- A tsp of ground cumin
- Two pounds of chopped carrots
- Two minced garlic cloves
- On diced sweet onion
- Two tbsp. of sesame oil

Method of preparation

In a cooking pot over medium heat, heat the sesame oil.

Include the minced garlic and diced onions and sauté them till they are translucent. Include the spices and carrots and cook them for three minutes. Pour in the water and broth and bring to boil. Reduce the heat gradually to a simmer to keep the carrots boiling in the broth. Cook for twenty minutes under the simmered heat.

Blend the cooked carrots in a blender or an immersion blender until they are partly smoothened. Into the blender, add the lime juice, siriracha syrup and the almond butter and blend to a smooth paste. Season the food with pepper and salt to taste. Serve immediately topped with chickpeas.

Super big salad with pickled red onions and basil ranch dressing

Salad Ingredients

- Seeds and nuts to sprinkle
- A diced avocado
- Vegetables and fruits of choice (for instance, a combination of pluots, julienned zucchinis, cherry tomatoes, sliced bell pepper, chopped red cabbage, and shredded carrots)
- Five handfuls of greens

Savory chickpeas ingredients

- A tbsp. of fresh lemon juice

- Two tbsp. of liquid aminos
- One and a half cups of cooked chickpeas

Roasted potatoes ingredients

- Pepper and salt to taste
- Some dashes of smoked paprika
- A few dashes of garlic powder
- Olive oil spray
- Two large red potatoes

Basil ranch dressing

- Half cup of packed fresh basil
- A quarter tsp of celery seeds
- A quarter tsp of dried dill
- Half tsp of onion powder
- Half tsp of garlic powder
- Half tsp of salt
- A tsp of agave syrup
- Two tbsp. of apple cedar vinegar
- Two tbsp. of fresh lemon juice
- Five tbsp. of water
- Half cup of raw cashew pre-soaked in hot water for two hours

Ingredients for pickled red onions

- A halved and thinly sliced red onion

- Four allspice berries
- A tsp of salt
- A tbsp. of agave syrup
- Half cup of apple cedar vinegar

Method of preparing the chickpeas

Put the chickpea in a heavy pan and cook over medium heat for a few minutes.

Include the liquid aminos and into the cooking chickpeas and stir. Cook for a few minutes till the chickpeas absorb all the liquid. Turn off the heat and let the chickpeas cool down before serving.

Method for preparing the roasted potatoes

Preheat your oven to 425F. Line a baking sheet with parchment paper. Put the chopped potatoes on the baking sheet. Spray on the potatoes with the olive oil. Add pepper salt, smoked paprika, and garlic powder, and toss them. Put the potatoes in the oven to cook for twenty minutes, halfway in the roasting toss the potatoes to cook evenly on all sides. When fully cooked, leave them to cool before including them in the salad.

Method for preparing picked red onions

Pour together the salt, agave syrup, and apple cedar vinegar in a jar. Include the all spice berries in the mixture and add the chopped red onions till fully covered in the liquid. Feel free to add more of the apple cedar vinegar (and shake well) if the onions are not fully submerged in the liquid. Refrigerate the contents in a tightly closed jar for at least four hours or alternatively leave it overnight.

Preparing the basil ranch dressing

In a food processor or high-speed blender, combine celery seeds, dill, onion powder, garlic powder, salt, agave syrup, apple cedar vinegar, lemon juice, water and cashews and process/blend to a smooth, consistent paste. Include the basil and process till even and smooth. Pour the blended mixture in to a tight container and keep chilled for 24hours or more but up to a maximum of 72hours.

Method of assembling the salad

Put together all the vegetables, fruits and greens and leave them in the fridge for five minutes. Once cooled, include the roasted potatoes and chickpeas and toss them to combine. Incorporate the avocado and toss the mixture to distribute evenly. Serve the salad into the individual bowls and generously drizzle on the dressing on top. Top with the pickled onions and sprinkle with more seeds and nuts.

It is now ready to go!

Summer plant-based food recipes

Sushi cups

- Half nori sheets
- Half tsp of red pepper flakes
- Half tsp of sea salt
- Two tsp of sesame oil
- Three tbsp. of liquid aminos
- A peeled and cubed cucumber
- A cored and cubed roma tomato
- A cubed small bell pepper

- Half avocado cut into cubes

Ingredients for preparing the rice cups

- A tbsp. of sesame oil
- A tbsp. of brown rice syrup
- A tbsp. of rice vinegar
- A tbsp. of liquid aminos
- Two cups of water
- A cupful of uncooked sushi rice or alternatively use short grain brown rice

Method

Clean the rice thoroughly and rain off the water.

Include the rice in a pot with two cups of water and bring to boil then reduce the heat to a simmer. Make sure the rice is still raging as you reduce the heat. Let the rice cook with a lid over for twenty minutes the turn off the heat and let it cool.

In a bowl include all the rice ingredients and combine them well then include them in the rice and mix.

Line a muffin tin with a parchment paper. Line the baking tin with another piece of paper that you will use to pull up the contents when cooked.

Include a table spoon to line up the muffin cups all the way from the bottom up then refrigerate for half an hour.

As for the filling, slice the bell peppers into cube- shapes and blanch them for two minutes then run cold water over then.

Combine all the marinade ingredients.

Dice the avocados, cucumber and tomato. Include then in a bowl along with all the vegetables. In this mixture pour in the marinade mixture and combine till evenly distributed.

Bring out the muffin cups and pill them out of the tin. Put them on a serving platter and include the vegetable mixture in them. Fill each cup and top them with vegan mayo or siracha sauce. Include a sprinkle of black sesame seeds on top.

Buffalo cauliflower pizza

Ingredients for the pizza sauce

- A quarter cup of wing sauce
- A tbsp. of vegan Worcestershire sauce
- Half can of tomato sauce

Ingredients for the buffalo cauliflower

- A tsp of garlic powder
- A cupful of vegan wing sauce
- Two tbsp. of olive oil
- A chopped medium sized cauliflower head

Ingredients for the pizza dough

- Salt
- Two tbsp. of olive oil
- Four cups of spelt flour

- A packet of active dry yeast
- A cupful of warm water

Ingredients for the vegan blue cheese dressing

- Salt
- Pepper
- A tbsp. of tahini
- Juice freshly squeezed from half a lemon
- A tsp of mustard powder
- One and half tsp of apple cedar vinegar
- Three tbsp. of almond milk
- Half can of artichoke heart
- Two tsp of artichoke liquid
- A pack of hemp tofu or half package of soy tofu

Method for preparing the vegan blue cheese dressing

In a blender, put together all the dressing ingredients and blend till they smoothen into a paste. Keep the processed mixture in a tight container and refrigerate.

Method for preparing the pizza crust

Pour in the dry yeast in warm water and let it sit for some minutes.

Include all the crust ingredients in a food processor and blend till the dough starts moving freely in the processor. Smear olive oil into a bowl and pour in the dough.

Keep the dough covered in the refrigerator for twelve hours.

Sprinkle on corn meal of flour on a flat surface and roll out the dough into the pizza shape.

The procedure of making a buffalo cauliflower

Preheat oven to 425F.

Toss the cauliflower with olive oil and bake in the oven in a baking sheet for fifteen minutes. Flip the florets to cook on both sides and replace in the oven cooking for ten more minutes. Mix the garlic powder and buffalo sauce in a bowl and stir.

When done, coat the cauliflower in the buffalo sauce and return to the oven to cook for another five minutes. Put together the sauce ingredients and mix them in a bowl. Place them aside.

In assembling the pizza, preheat your oven to 500F. Preheat the baking sheet or pizza stone in the oven for seven minutes as you work on preparing the pizza for baking. Sprinkle the pizza with the sauce covering it wholly. Place the cooked buffalo cauliflower on top. Put the pizza in the oven and let it cook for ten minutes. It should attain a crispy feel to it hen done.

When done, take it out of the oven and sprinkle on the blue cheese dressing topping with the cilantro.

Barbecue beans

Ingredients

- Three chopped scallions
- Half cup of chopped pickles
- A cup full of chopped and cooked collard greens
- A cupful of barbecue sauce

- Two cups of barbecued beans
- Warm tortilla chips
- A can of diced chili -tomatoes
- A quarter tsp of onion granules
- Three quarter teaspoons of sea salt
- Two tbsp. of nutritional yeast
- Three tbsp. of tapioca starch
- Three tbsp. of chopped and roasted peppers
- Half cup of plain vegan yoghurt
- Three quarter cups of unsweetened non-dairy milk
- A cupful of mashed silken tofu

Method of preparation

Put the onions, salt, yeast, tapioca, red pepper, yoghurt, milk, and tofu in a blender and blend to a smooth paste.

In a medium pot, pour in the blended mixture and bring to boil.

Include the diced tomatoes into the mixture and stir. Reduce the heat to a simmer. Cook the mixture to thicken and check if the tapioca is well done before turning off the heat.

In a toaster oven, separately warm the barbecue sauce, warm the barbecue beans and warm the chips.

Boil or steam the collards and completely drain off the water. Slice the scallions and pickles.

Put the tortilla chips into layers and put the barbecue beans on top. Sprinkle barbecue sauce on top, add the scallions, pickles, collards and the cheese sauce.

Serve and enjoy immediately.

Baked spinach and bulgur veggie balls

Ingredients

- Spices of choice
- One third cupful of hulled raw sunflowers
- A quarter cupful of pitted olives
- One third cup of cooked chickpeas
- Three a half ounce of fresh spinach
- One and a third cupful of bulgur
- Three eggs of chia eggs or three tbsp of soaked chia (presoaked for ten minutes)

Method

Put the bulgur in water and let it soak for ten minutes. When soaked, drain the water and rinse it.

Slice the spinach into thin strips.

Preheat your oven to 320F.

Put together the ingredients in a large bowl and mix. Make medium sized balls from the mixture. Moisten your hands to prevent them from sticking on. Place the vegie balls on a baking tray lined with parchment paper. Cook for half an hour. The vegie balls should roll freely off the baking sheet when done.

You can have the ball alongside herbs and pasta.

Cornbread pizza cake

Ingredients for the cornbread

- Two tbsp. of maple syrup
- Three tbsp. of unsalted sundried roughly chopped tomatoes
- Two tbsp. of diced jalapenos and more for topping
- Oil
- Half tsp of salt
- Three tsp of baking powder
- A tbsp. of apple cedar vinegar
- A cupful of unsweetened almond milk
- Three tbsp. of water
- A tbsp. of chia seeds
- One third cup of apple sauce
- One and a half cup of cornmeal

Ingredients for the cake

- Three batches of sundried tomatoes
- Fire roasted corn
- A diced red onion
- Grilled red bell peppers
- A sliced avocado
- A pizza sauce
- One third cup of vegan nacho cheese
- Three quarter cups of guacamole

- 57ounces of oil-free refried beans

Method of preparation

Preheat your oven to 425F.

Mix chia seeds with water, whisk the mixture and set aside to form a chia egg.

Combine the almond milk with apple cedar vinegar and set aside for five minutes.

Combine salt, baking powder, and corn flour in a bowl. Include the jalapenos and the sundried tomatoes and combine again.

To the dry mixture, add the chia egg, milk mixture, and apple sauce and mix without getting it overdone.

Line a rounded baking pan with a parchment paper and pour in the mixture to the top of the pan.

Bake the bread in the oven for fifteen minutes till well done, and the edges turn brown. Test if cooked using a toothpick.

Method for making the pizza cake

Layer the cornbread with nacho cheese and refried beans. Include another layer of the cornbread topped with guacamole. Place on another layer topped with fire roasted corn, diced red onions, the grilled red peppers, sliced avocado, and the pizza sauce.

Slice the pizza and serve with a lime slice on the side.

Kimchi zucchini pasta

Ingredients for preparing the zucchini pasta

- Thinly sliced nori sheets

- Thinly sliced green onion or chives
- A quarter cup of roughly chopped kimchi and extra for topping
- A pinch of salt
- A light drizzle of sesame oil
- One and a half pounds of zucchinis

Ingredients for the cream sauce

- Some cracks of black pepper
- Half tsp of salt
- Half tsp of tamari
- One and half tsp of toasted sesame oil
- Four tbsp. of lemon juice
- Two tsp of kimchi liquid
- Three quarter cups of vegan kimchi
- A cupful of cashews

Method for preparing the kimchi cream sauce

Soak cashews in water for at least four hours. When ready to use them, drain the water and rinse them in clean water.

Pour all the sauce ingredients in the blender and blend to a smooth paste. When using the regular blender, add some water to the mixture to help in blending. For a high-speed blender, use the tamper to help the mixture form into cream.

Method for preparing the zucchini pasta

Use a spiralizer to make the zucchini noodles.

Split the noodles to make them shorter and more comfortable to eat.

Place the noodles in a bowl and add a pinch of salt and sprinkle on with the sesame oil. Combine the mixture by tossing and let it sit for three minutes.

Assembling the components

Slice the nori into thin sheets. Chop the green onions or chives thinly. Chop the kimchi roughly. Use the kimchi sauce to toss the zucchini and ensure they are well covered in the sauce. Include the roughly chopped kimchi and mix. Place the pasta on a plate and top with the nori sheets, green onion slices or chive slices, and include the extra kimchi you had reserved for topping.

Chickpea quinoa-cake

Ingredients for the cake

- Thinly sliced fresh scallions for garnishing
- Fresh black pepper
- Nutritional yeast flakes
- A quarter tsp of paprika
- A quarter tsp of paprika
- A quarter tsp of mustard powder
- A quarter tsp of cayenne pepper
- A tbsp. of flaxseed meal in three tbsp. of hot water
- Two tbsp. of vegan mayo
- A quarter tsp of fresh minced parsley
- A tbsp. of fresh lemon juice
- A tsp of vegan Worcestershire sauce

- Two tbsp. of finely diced onions
- A quarter cup of finely diced celery
- A quarter cup of finely diced red pepper
- A cupful of shredded zucchini
- A cupful of cooked quinoa
- A can of low sodium chickpeas

Ingredients for roast pepper cashew cream sauce

- Fresh black pepper to taste
- A dash of cayenne pepper
- Four tbsp. of unsweetened almond milk
- Two tbsp. of water
- A minced garlic clove
- A quarter diced and roasted pepper
- A tsp. of horse radish
- A tsp of Dijon mustard
- Four tbsp. of lemon juice
- Half tsp of dill weeds
- A half cup of cashews soaked in water for four hours

Method of preparation for the cashew cream sauce

Put half cup of cashews in water in a bowl till fully covered for at least four hours. When ready to use them drain off the water and rinse them in clean water. Put the cashews in a blender along with the other ingredients and blend to a smooth paste. Keep the cashew cream chilled till serving time.

Method of preparation for the cake

Preheat your oven to 375F.

Follow the packaging instructions in preparing the quinoa and ensure it has fully absorbed all the liquid. After it is cooked, let it cool first before using it. Mix three tablespoons of hot water with the tablespoon of flaxseed and let it sit for a few minutes.

Drain the garbanzo beans off the water and rinse thoroughly in clean room temperature water. Partly mash the beans in a mixing bowl. When well mashed, include the rest of the cake ingredients and combine.

With a cooking spray, coat a non-sticky cooking pan. Scoop the mixture into each muffin cup to closely fill. Push the batter down firmly into the cup by use of the scooping spoon. Sprinkle on the dough in the baking pan with nutritional yeast flakes. Bake cake in the oven for forty minutes. It should come off golden brown and crispy on the top. Give the cakes five minutes to cool down the run a sharp object thought he edges to detach it from the tin.

Place the cooked cupcakes on a service platter and sprinkle on the cashew sauce on top. Garnish with chopped chives or scallions.

You can serve the cake with a salad of choice.

Roasted ratatouille spaghetti

Ingredients for the sauce

- Fresh parsley for garnishing
- Pepper and salt
- A minced garlic clove

- A tbsp. of maple syrup or agave nectar
- Half tbsp. of tomato paste
- One and a half tbsp. of miso paste

Ingredients for the ratatouille and pasta

- A quarter of a large onion diced into pieces
- A quarter of a butternut squash
- A can of tomatoes (preferably 114ounces)
- Four ounces of gluten-free spaghetti

Method of preparation

Preheat your oven to 450F.

In a baking tray, toss the onions, butternut squash and eggplant with pepper and salt put the mixture in the oven and bake for ten minutes till they are softened and caramelized.

In preparing the pasta, put some salt in water in a pot and bring to boil. Follow the instruction on the package on how to prepare your pasta. When cooked, drain the water and keep aside. The pasta should be soft but not soggy. Run through cold water and drain immediately to prevent the pasta from sticking on each other.

When the baking vegetables are well cooked, pour them into a bowl and set aside. In a cooking pot include the agave, garlic, tomato paste, miso, and the canned tomatoes. Include some pasta water in the sauce and cook under low heat.

When done, pour your pasta into a bowl. Include warm vegetables in the bowl and toss. Pour in your warm sauce and mix. Season the pasta with pepper and salt to taste and garnish with fresh parsley.

Fall plant food recipes

Pumpkin spice pancakes

Ingredients

- A cupful of whole meal pastry flour
- A quarter cup of cinnamon
- A tsp of pumpkin pie spice
- A pinch of salt
- Half tsp of baking soda
- A tsp of baking powder
- A tbsp. of agave or maple syrup
- Three tbsp. of brown sugar
- Half tsp of pure vanilla extract
- A tbsp. of vegan butter
- One third of a cupful of pumpkin puree
- A tbsp. of white vinegar or lemon juice
- A cupful of unsweetened vanilla almond milk

Method of preparation

Preheat your electric griddle to 350F. You can alternatively use a large skillet on medium low heat. A drop of oil on the skillet should not burn or evaporate immediately.

Pour together the lemon juice or vinegar in a bowl and the almond milk and stir. Set aside the mixture for five minutes. In the curdled mixture, include the vanilla extract, brown sugar, maple syrup, pumpkin puree and the vegan butter and combine.

In a sifter, combine the spices, salt, baking powder, baking soda, and flour and sift the mixture over the mixture of the wet ingredients. Combine the mixture thoroughly. Balance the thickness of the batter using the almond milk and flour to attain a desirable thickness. Let the mixture rest for up to ten minutes or less.

Spray on your griddle or skillet with oil. Pour a quarter cup of the mixture on the hot griddle or skillet. When the pancake dries up on the surface, bubbles on the top and the edges start detaching form the hot surface, flip on the pancake to cook on the other side. Cook the other side a few minutes longer them remove the pancake and place it in a warmed plate. Repeat the same process for the remaining batter. You should come up with approximately six pancakes as per the measurements in the recipe.

Top the cooked pancakes with the pumpkin pie spice, vegan butter, and maple syrup.

You can leave the pancakes covered and microwave to eat the following day. Or enjoy while still warm.

Vegan broccoli and cheese soup

Ingredients for preparing the soup

- One and a half tsp of chickpea miso
- Freshly ground black pepper to taste

- Half tsp of sea salt
- One and a half tsp of freshly squeezed lemon juice
- Two and a half tbsp. of water
- A quarter tsp of cayenne pepper
- Two tbsp. of nutritional yeast
- Three cups of low sodium vegetable broth
- One and a half cups of chopped Yukon gold potatoes
- Six cups of chopped broccoli florets
- A cupful of chopped celery
- Three minced medium garlic cloves
- One diced medium onion
- A tbsp. of extra virgin olive oil

Ingredients for the preparing the Cheese Sauce

- Half tsp of white wine vinegar
- A medium garlic clove
- Half tsp of fine salt
- One and a half tsp of fresh lemon juice
- Two and a half tsp of water
- Two tbsp. of refined grape seed oil or coconut oil
- Two tbsp. of nutritional yeast
- One third of a cup of peeled and diced carrots
- One and a quarter cups of peeled and diced red or yellow potatoes

Topping ingredients

- Freshly minced parsley
- Sweet or smoked paprika
- Pan-fried garlic croutons

Method of preparation

For the cheese sauce:

In a medium pot over high heat bring the carrots and potatoes to boil. When boiled lower the heat to medium until they are well cooked and softened. The process should take up to fifteen minutes. When cooked drain foo the water.

In a high-speed blender, blend the vinegar, garlic, salt, lemon juice, water, oil, and nutritional yeast and set the blended mixture aside. After a few minutes include the boiled carrots and potatoes and blend the mixture to a smooth sauce.

Preparation for the soup:

Chop the soup ingredients including the potatoes, broccoli, celery, garlic, and onions and set them aside.

Fry the garlic and onions in oil over medium heat. Cook them for up to five minutes in a large pot. Stir they cook when they translucent and add the potatoes, broccoli, and celery and sauté for five minutes. Include the pepper, salt, lemon juice, cayenne pepper, nutritional yeast, and the broth. Stir and cover the pot. Let the food cook over medium heat for fifteen minutes. When the potatoes are softened, turn off the heat and let the food sit for ten minutes. Include the miso in the pot and stir.

In a blender, bend all the soup in batches till in smoothens and pour it back to the pot. Include half of the sauce to the pot and stir in. The other half of the sauce will be used for garnishing. If need be, add more seasoning.

Serve the soup into the individual bowls and swirl a tsp of the cheese sauce over the bowls. Top the soup with parsley, paprika, and pan-fried garlic croutons.

Vegan pumpkin ravioli

Ingredients for the white wine sage butter sauce

- Ground black pepper
- Sea salt
- A quarter cup of white wine
- Two tbsp. of roughly chopped fresh
- A quarter cup of finely chopped onions
- A tbsp. of vegan butter

Pumpkin cheese filing

- Half tsp of ground black pepper or white pepper
- A tsp of nutmeg
- A tsp of dried basil
- A tsp of sage
- A tsp of sea salt
- One third cup of low sodium vegetable stock
- Three garlic cloves

- A tbsp. of lemon juice
- A tbsp. of tomato paste
- One third cup of nutritional yeast
- One third cup of raw cashews pre-soaked in hot water for twenty minutes
- A cupful of pumpkin puree

Ingredients for the dough

- Half tsp of sea salt
- A cupful of water
- One and a half cups of whole wheat flour
- One and a half cups of all-purpose flour

Method for preparation

Mix the flour ingredients and salt thoroughly in a bowl. Combine with the water by creating a depression in the middle and pouring in the cupful of water. Use a wooden spoon to mix the flour with water. When combined, pour out on a floured flat surface. Use your hands to mix the dough by pressing and folding it. When the dough becomes less sticky, roll it up and put in back into the bowl covered to rest.

Remove the cashews from the water and wash them with clean cold water. In a high-speed blender, blend together all the filling ingredients to a smooth paste. Avoid adding more water to the ingredients as they blend. Put the blended mixture into the fridge as you work-on the ravioli.

Work on the dough in halves. Place the dough on a floured surface and roll it into a very thin shape. Use a squared 4inch cookie cutter to draw out as many pieces as the dough can give.

Place the cut-out pieces on a floured baking sheet and cover it as you work on the remaining pieces. Place a tsp of the filling on half the cut outs and use a wet finger to moisten the edges.

Place another piece on top and join them by pressing them together. You can freeze them by keeping them floured and having a baking sheet between them as you store.

In a pot of water boil the ravioli until they surface on the water. You can boil in batches each taking up to three minutes. When they are done, heat a pan over medium heat. Fry the onions in the butter till they soften. Include sage and stir. Let it cook for a few minutes. Put in the ravioli and cook them evenly on both sides. Season them with black pepper and salt. The ravioli should cook along with the onions and sage for two minutes then add white wine vinegar and let it cook for another three minutes. If you have too many ravioli to cook, cook a few at a time to avoid overloading the pan. In the serving bowl include the remaining filling then place the raviolis on top.

Winter recipes

Vegetable foil packets

Ingredients

- Four tbsp. of extra virgin olive oil

- Four garlic heads
- One large red onion 50 grams of baby potatoes
- Three medium carrots
- A medium zucchini

Ingredients for the spice mix

- Three quarter tsp of salt
- Two tbsp. of marjoram
- A tsp of sweet paprika
- A quarter tsp of black pepper
- A tsp of dried garlic

Method of preparation

Preheat the oven to 400F

Remove the outer cover of the garlic. Chop onions into rings. Quarter the baby potatoes. Peel off the carrots and chop them. Slice the zucchini into medium pieces. Put all the vegetables in a bowl leaving aside the garlic. Sprinkle on olive oil and mix to ensure all pieces are coated.

Combine all the spice ingredients in a bowl and sprinkle the spice mix on the vegetables toss the vegetables to ensure the spices are widely spread. Share the vegetables in four foils. Place the garlic on the spice mix to take in all the spices and include them in the middle of the foil. Let each foil have a garlic clove in it. When done, transfer them into a baking tray wrapping them with the foil. Let the vegetables bake for up to 35 minutes.

Grilled eggplant

Ingredients for the jerk barbecue sauce

- Reserved marinade
- Half cup of barbecue sauce

Ingredients

- Two tbsp. of coconut
- One large eggplant cut in two-inch pieces

Marinade ingredients

- Two tbsp. of mirin
- A tbsp. of lime juice
- Two tbsp. of soy sauce
- Two tbsp. coconut sugar
- Four tbsp. of Jamaican jerk seasoning

Method of preparation

Put together the marinade ingredients and give them up to three hours to set. Place the eggplant chops on skewers and sprinkle them with melted coconut oil. Heat up the grill to 400F and let the eggplants grill for five minutes on either side.

Mix the dipping sauce ingredients and serve them alongside the eggplant skewers.

Black bean burgers

Ingredients

- Half cup of dried breadcrumbs
- Half cup sun-dried tomatoes in oil
- Two tbsp. of olive oil
- Half medium red onion
- A tsp of paprika
- One and a half tsp of cumin
- Half tsp of salt
- A can of black beans
- Two flax eggs (two tbsp. of flax seeds dissolved in six tbsp. of water)
- Half cup of rolled oats

Method of preparation

Drain the black beans and mash them using your clean hands, fork or a masher.

Chop the sundried tomatoes and the red onions and include them in a bowl. Include the olive oil, paprika, cumin, salt, and flax eggs. Add the breadcrumbs in bits as you mix till you achieve a firm mixture.

Use your hands to form burger patties of the mixture. You can fry the burger in some oil in a pan or grill on a barbecue grill. Let each side cook for five minutes on each side. Serve the burger as you prefer it. You can serve with lettuce, tomatoes, and a ban.

Chapter 5:

Grocery List for Plant Based Foods

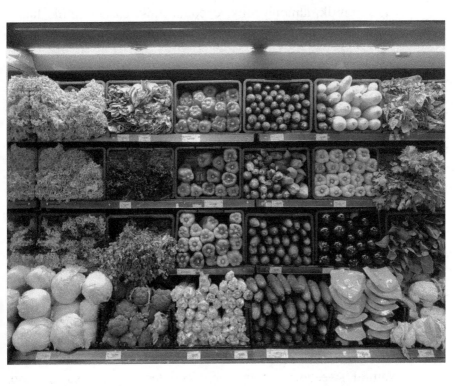

When shopping for your kitchen there are certain foods you need to look for in the store and they are as follows;

- Fruits; this includes all types of fruits. Be it fresh or frozen.
- Vegetables; this refers to the canned, frozen, and fresh vegetables.
- Legumes; this includes all legumes ranging from soy products (soy milk, soy protein, edamame, tempeh and tofu) to all beans and lentils.

- All herbs and spices, vinegar, nutritional yeast, baking soda, and baking powder
- Dairy alternatives; such as dairy free milk, coconut yoghurt, cashew milk, almond milk, coconut milk, cashew milk, hemp milk, rice milk, soy milk, oat milk, non-dairy cheese (cashew cheese)
- Processed dairy alternatives; vegan ice cream, earth balance butter, coconut cream, chocolate soy, cheese slices, mozzarella or cheddar style shreds, vegan cream cheese, and vegan sour cream.
- Whole grains and whole grain products. It also Includes whole grain flour.
- Lightly processed foods for instance cereals.
- Seeds and nuts, Peanut products, nut butter such as peanut butter, cashew butter, and almond butter, seed butter such as sunflower seed butter and tahini butter.
- Natural sweeteners; they include dates, organic sugar cane, stevia, molasses, maple syrup, coconut sugar, and agave syrup.
- Avoid purchasing; honey, gelatin, fish, meat, poultry, dairy milk, cheese, eggs, cream and butter.
- Condiments; vinegar (red wine, balsamic, apple cedar, white wine), sauerkraut, nutritional yeast, sweet chili sauce, organic ketchup, salsa, mustard, miso paste, soy sauce/tamari, green curry paste, red curry paste, and coconut milk.

Conclusion

Thank you for making it through to the end of *Plant based cookbook*, let's hope it was informative and able to provide you with all of the tools you need to achieve your goals whatever they may be.

The next step is trying out the different recipes outlined in the book. As we have seen in the book, there are many advantages of adapting to plant-based foods. Generally, it is the best way of a healthy life. If you are battling with weight challenges why not try out the low-calorie recipes? You don't have to go fully blown vegan rather every once in a while, killing those meat cravings the right way. Over time you will realize the benefits of eating plant foods.

If you have been through this book you certainly enjoy being in the kitchen. Experiment with different foods and create your own recipes. Check out other recipe books and borrow ideas from them. You don't have to be strict with the methods given in the book: instead create your own from the ideas you attained from this book. As you enjoy the recipes, share out with your family and friends and let every meal tell a tale.

Finally, if you found this book useful in any way, a review on Amazon is always appreciated!

CPSIA information can be obtained
at www.ICGtesting.com
Printed in the USA
LVHW100732061120
670424LV00042B/226